ECG Workbook

ECG Workbook

Rohan Jayasinghe

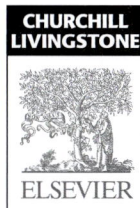

CHURCHILL
LIVINGSTONE

ELSEVIER

Sydney Edinburgh London New York Philadelphia St Louis Toronto

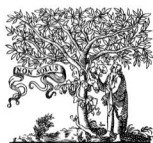

ELSEVIER

Churchill Livingstone
is an imprint of Elsevier

Elsevier Australia. ACN 001 002 357
(a division of Reed International Books Australia Pty Ltd)
Tower 1, 475 Victoria Avenue, Chatswood, NSW 2067

National Library of Australia Cataloguing-in-Publication entry

Author: Jayasinghe, S. Rohan.

Title: ECG workbook / Rohan Jayasinghe.

ISBN: 9780729541091 (pbk.)

Subjects: Electrocardiography–Interpretation.
             Heart–Diseases–Diagnosis.

Dewey Number: 616.1207547

Publisher: Luisa Cecotti
Developmental Editor: Neli Bryant
Project Coordinator: Karthikeyan Murthy and Natalie Hamad
Edited by Brenda Hamilton
Proofread by Gabrielle Challis
Cover and internal design by Georgette Hall
Index by Robert Swanson
Typeset by Toppan Best-set Premedia Limited
Printed in China Translation & Printing Services Ltd

Contents

Preface

Many books are aimed at helping clinicians and students with ECG competency, but none of these books focuses on the clinical context related to the ECG. I always emphasise to my trainees that we do not treat ECGs but patients. So I decided to create this book in which the reader is guided through the ECG to make a clinical diagnosis and decide on the appropriate management.

ECG Workbook provides an easy but systematic algorithm to follow when attempting to read an ECG. The exercises are aimed at training the reader to practise this algorithm repeatedly with different ECGs. The real-life clinical synopsis essentially links the ECG findings to the patient's clinical context. This information guides the reader to make a clinical diagnosis with the help of the ECG findings, and then to decide on the optimal treatment or management plan.

ECG Workbook attempts to train the reader on how to systematically and accurately read and interpret ECGs in the real-life clinical or ward setting, where multiple abnormalities can manifest in the one ECG. The reader is trained to stratify the significance of the ECG findings based on clinical urgency and the relevance to the patient's active pathology.

It is hoped that by completing this workbook the reader will gain the required mastery to use ECG as a clinical diagnostic tool effectively and to make suitable management decisions with confidence.

Rohan Jayasinghe

Foreword

Professor Rohan Jayasinghe's *ECG Workbook* has already proved popular with medical students as its case-based, user-friendly format complements other currently available material on ECG interpretation.

As an active interventional cardiologist, Professor Jayasinghe interprets ECGs in a variety of clinical circumstances, such as in the catheter laboratory, at the bedside and at the clinic, all of which add to the value of the workbook for the student. As the author of other respected books for (undergraduate and postgraduate) trainees in medicine, and a teacher of clinical students, he brings the perspective of modern teaching methods to *ECG Workbook*.

The world of clinical cardiology is changing and progressing at an increasing rate, so this workbook not only trains the student of today but prepares them to think along evidence-based lines which will help these clinicians of the future keep up with, and possibly even contribute to, the progress of this important part of medical practice.

Ian Hamilton-Craig

MB, BS (Adel), PhD (McMaster), FRACP, FCSANZ, FLS (Lond)

Professor of Preventive Cardiology

Griffith University School of Medicine

Southport, Queensland, Australia

Acknowledgements

I wish to acknowledge the following people for their support in the conception of *ECG Workbook*:

- The Cardiac Scientists at the Gold Coast Hospital who helped, including Terri Costello, Carolyn Brown, Beth VanderWall, and the Director of Clinical Measurement, Vivek Kulkarni.
- The very supportive team at Elsevier, including Sophie Kaliniecki who saw the potential of this venture and Neli Bryant who guided the process.
- My wife Hanna for her critical input and practical suggestions.
- My parents for their constant encouragement.

The author

Rohan Jayasinghe MBBS (Honours First Class)(Sydney), MSpM, PhD, FRACP, FCSANZ, MBA (Newcastle)

Professor of Cardiology, School of Medicine, Griffith University, Queensland, Director of Cardiac Services/Cardiology, Gold Coast Hospital, Queensland

Reviewers

Lucy Cho MBBS, MIPH, BA (Sydney)
Resident, The Wollongong Hospital, Wollongong, New South Wales

Stewart Mann DM (Oxon), FRCP, FRACP, FCSANZ
Associate Professor of Cardiovascular Medicine, University of Otago, Wellington, New Zealand

Jason Verden MBBS
Senior Resident Medical Officer Critical Care, The Canberra Hospital, Australian Capital Territory

Selina Watchorn MBBS, BNursing, BArts
The Canberra Hospital, Australian National University, Australian Capital Territory

SECTION 1
BASICS OF THE ECG

WHY THE ECG?

Why is the electrocardiogram (ECG) important? It provides a composite snapshot of the electrical activity of the heart from several different projections or directions. These projections focus on the different regions of the heart. Electrical activity of the heart may give important information about cardiac health and pathology.

Thus the ECG provides very important and time-critical information related to cardiac function, cardiac health and cardiac pathology. When the patient is connected to an ECG monitor, this information is available in real time.

GENERATION AND REGULATION OF THE CARDIAC CYCLE

Cardiac muscle cells are able to generate electrical potentials by spontaneous depolarisation. This causes the heart to contract. The heart also has the ability to regulate these impulses. The ability of the heart to generate and regulate its own electrical impulses is called automaticity. The electrical impulses are conducted along cardiac cells via the gap junctions that exist between cells (Fig 1.1).

The rate at which cardiac muscle contracts is determined by the region of the heart that generates the impulses (the node). However, the heart is also subject to autonomic nervous system control and affected by certain hormone levels in the circulation. Sympathetic drive accelerates the heart rate while the vagal or parasympathetic drive slows it down. Adrenergic drive will accelerate the heart.

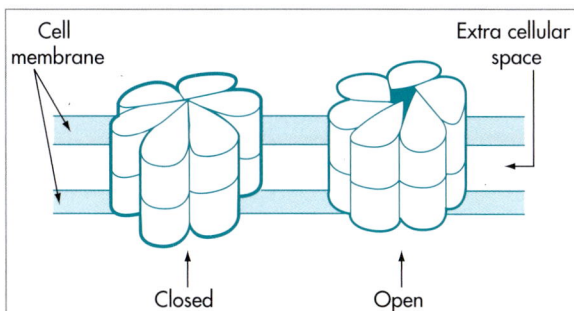

Figure 1.1 A gap junction

CARDIAC CONDUCTION SYSTEM

Under normal circumstances, cardiac rhythm is generated by the sinoatrial (SA) node located in the superior–lateral aspect of the right atrium. Impulse generated in the SA node leads to contraction of the atria. This impulse is carried along the atrial tissue to the atrioventricular (AV) node located in the lower region of the right atrium close to its junction with the ventricles. The conductivity of the AV node is slower, so it *can* act as a filter to prevent rapid (uncontrolled) rates conducting through to the ventricles. This delay of the conduction at the level of the AV node is required to allow adequate time for the ventricles to fill during diastole.

If the SA node fails to fire, the AV node can take over the cardiac rhythm (impulse) generation but at a much slower rate. From the AV node the impulse is conducted via the bundle of His (a bundle of conductive fibres) to the ventricles. Within the ventricle the bundle of His divides into the right and left conduction tissue bundles that carry the impulse to the respective ventricles. The left bundle has two branches, anterior and posterior.

CARDIAC CONDUCTION SYSTEM IN DETAIL

This system helps to generate cardiac electrical impulses that give rise to the cardiac electric potential, which spreads through the entire myocardium leading to its contraction and relaxation in a sequential manner (Fig 1.2). This is called the cardiac cycle.

- SA node is the collection of cardiac conduction cells with the fastest intrinsic rate of depolarisation or impulse generation. SA node acts as the primary and dominant signal generator. It is located in the superior–lateral aspect of the right atrial free wall (on the opposite side to the interatrial septum). It normally depolarises at a rate of 60–100 impulses (beats) per minute. SA node starts the cardiac cycle and triggers atrial contraction.

- AV node is the collection of cardiac conduction cells located in the lower edge of the interatrial septum. It has a slower rate of conduction, so it causes a delay in the conduction of electrical impulse from the atrium to the ventricle, thus acting as a 'rate filter'. This delay allows the required time for the filling of the ventricular

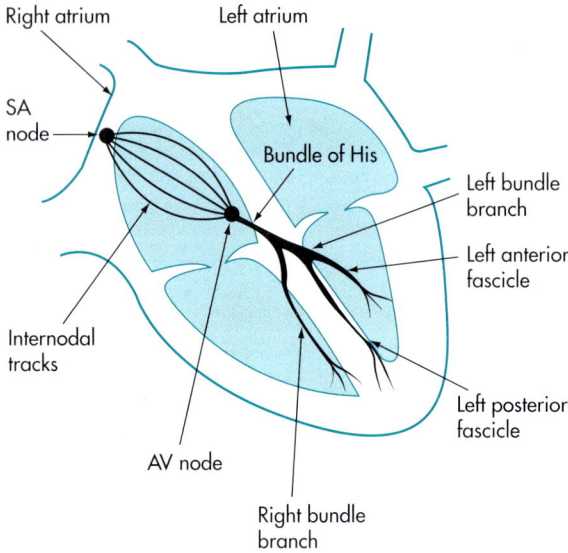

Figure 1.2 The cardiac conduction system

Phase 0 = depolarisation (Na⁺ enters the cell)
Phase 1 = repolarisation
Phase 2 = corresponds to ST segment
Phase 3 = repolarisation corresponds to T wave
Phase 4 = resting potential

Figure 1.3 Cardiac action potential

cavities with blood during ventricular diastole that coincides with atrial systole.

- The His–Purkinje system is the section of the cardiac conduction system that carries the electrical impulse from the AV node to the two electricity conduits (bundle branches) supplying the two ventricles: the right bundle branch and the left bundle branch. The current is carried to the right ventricle by one branch and to the left ventricle by two branches or conduits called fascicles created by the division of the left bundle branch. These two divisions are called left anterior and posterior fascicles of the left bundle branch.

- Defects or pathologies of the conduction system can lead to bradyarrhythmias and conduction abnormalities. These include sinus bradycardia, other bradyarrhythmias, heart-blocks and bundle branch blocks.

BASIC PHYSIOLOGY OF THE CARDIAC CONDUCTION SYSTEM

Cardiac action potential is the graphic representation of the changes in the electrical potential that take place across the cardiac muscle cell membrane. The action potential starts with the depolarisation of the cell membrane and finishes with the repolarisation of it prior to the next cycle of depolarisation.

- Phase 0 — Depolarisation is caused by a rapid flow of Na⁺ and Ca⁺⁺ ions (current) from

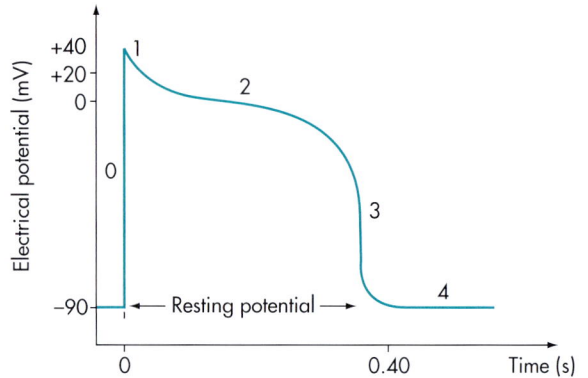

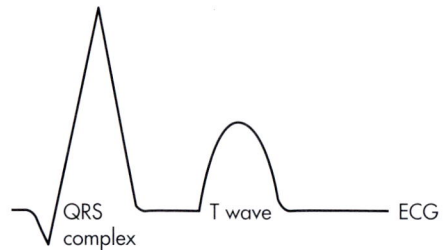

outside the cell across the membrane to the inside of the cell via ion-specific channels. This depolarisation commences at a trigger potential of 65 mV. Depolarisation is shown in the graph (Fig 1.3) as the first upstroke: this is 'Phase 0' of the action potential.

- Phase 1 — In the next sequence the Na⁺ channels rapidly close, which stops the inward flow of the Na⁺ ions across the membrane. Now begins a rapid flow of K⁺ ions from inside the cell to the outside via open K⁺ channels. This leads to a rapid repolarisation of the cell membrane: this segment is called Phase 1 of the action potential.

- Phase 2 — Slow Ca⁺⁺ channels open and allow the inward flow of Ca⁺⁺ ions that persists with the outward flow of K⁺ ions. This flow of cations (positive ions) in opposite directions slows down the repolarisation process, hence Phase 2 is seen as the plateau phase.

- Phase 3 — The Ca⁺⁺ channels close but the K⁺ channels remain open with the outward flow of K⁺ ions. This segment signifies a rapid repolarisation.

- Phase 4 — In this phase the resting electrical potential of the cell membrane is restored. There is a correction of the excess Na^+ ions accumulated inside the cell and the excess K^+ ions accumulated outside the cell by the activation of Na^+/K^+ exchange channels.

Note in Figure 1.3 how cardiac action potential and the relevant changes in the cell membrane potential correlate with the ECG waveform and the cardiac electrical complex or the PQRS complex.

THE RATE, SCALE AND CALIBRATION

The first step in reading an ECG involves determining the rate. Rate calculation (Fig 1.4(a)) is dependent upon the scale and the calibration used in recording the ECG. The scale determines the distance and the voltage represented by the

grid on which the ECG is recorded (Fig 1.4(b)). Calibration is the speed at which the ECG is recorded.

WILLIAM EINTHOVEN AND THE EINTHOVEN TRIANGLE

William Einthoven, a Dutch physician and physiologist, described and developed a way to detect and record cardiac electrical activity from the surface of the body for which he was awarded the Nobel Prize in Medicine in 1924. The letters P, QRS and T, used to define the various components of an ECG tracing, were first used by Einthoven.

The electrical activity in the heart was initially recorded with electrodes placed between the left and right arm and the left leg. The voltage and its direction between two electrodes are represented

(a) Measuring the rate of rhythm of an ECG

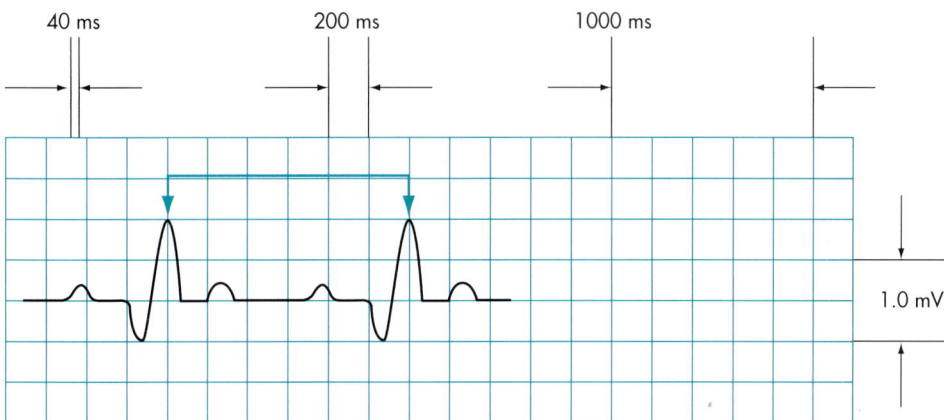

(b) ECG paper grid

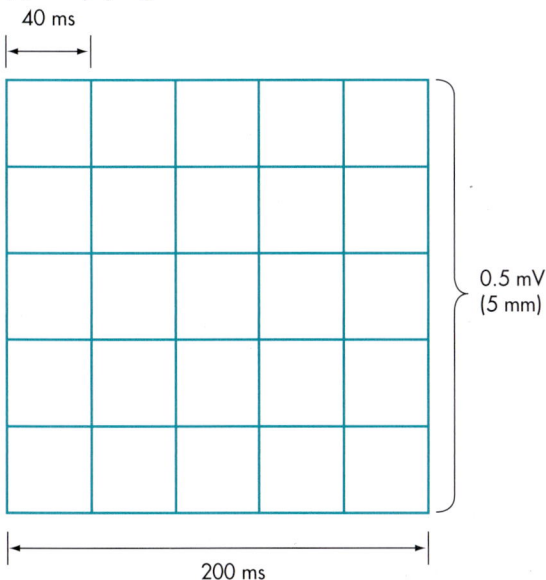

Figure 1.4 (a) Determining the rate of the rhythm of an ECG; (b) ECG paper grid and measurements

Standard leads   I   II   III

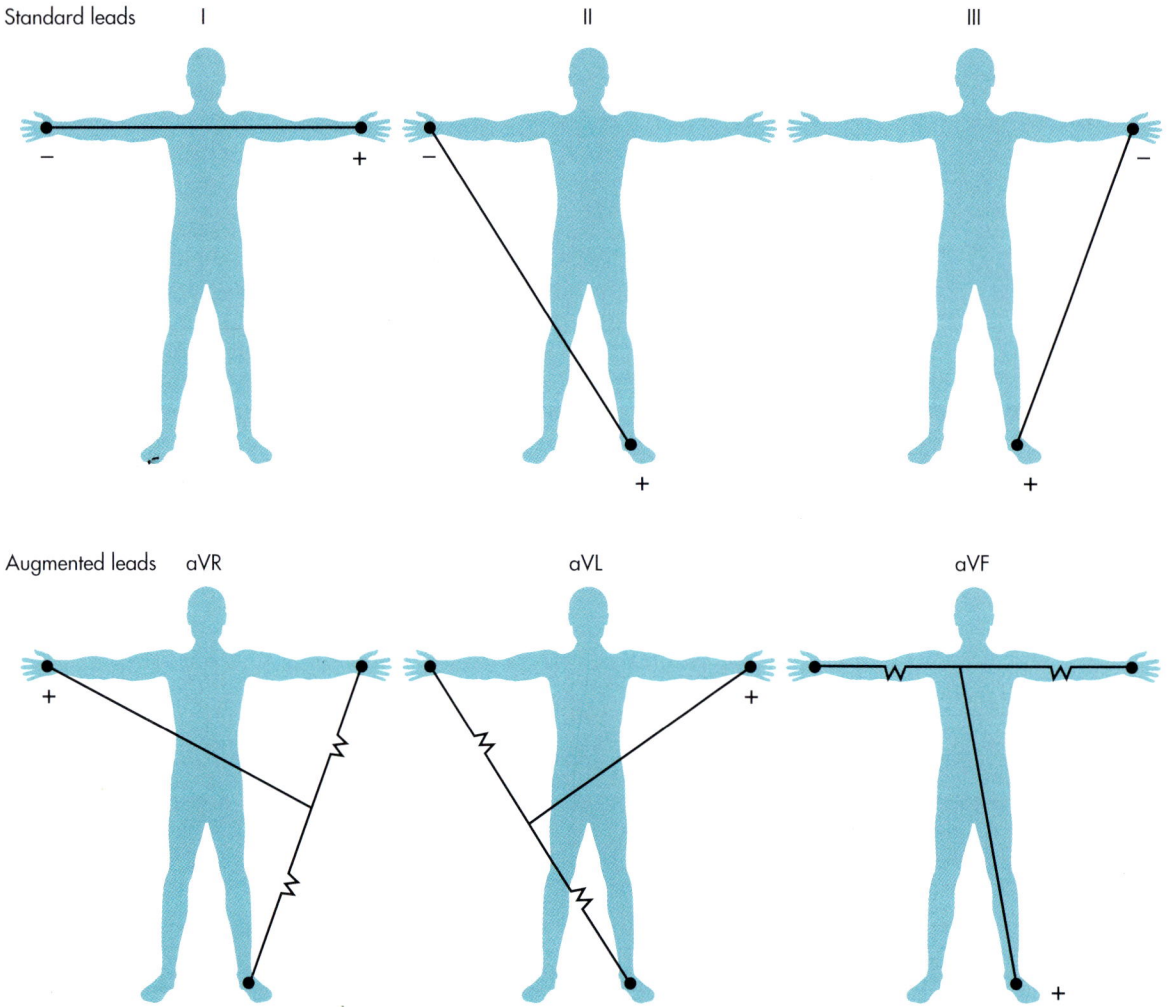

Figure 1.5 Limb leads

Augmented leads   aVR   aVL   aVF

by a lead. Thus the space between the electrodes placed in the limbs where the voltage is measured is called a limb lead.

The three standard limb leads (Fig 1.5) are:

- Lead I — between left and right arms
- Lead II — between the right arm and the left leg
- Lead III — between the left arm and the left leg.

The inverted triangle created by the three limb leads connecting the three limb electrodes is called Einthoven's triangle (Fig 1.6). The heart, situated at the centre of this triangle, thus becomes the electrically neutral point. The electrical axis of the heart or the direction along which the current is flowing is determined using this triangle.

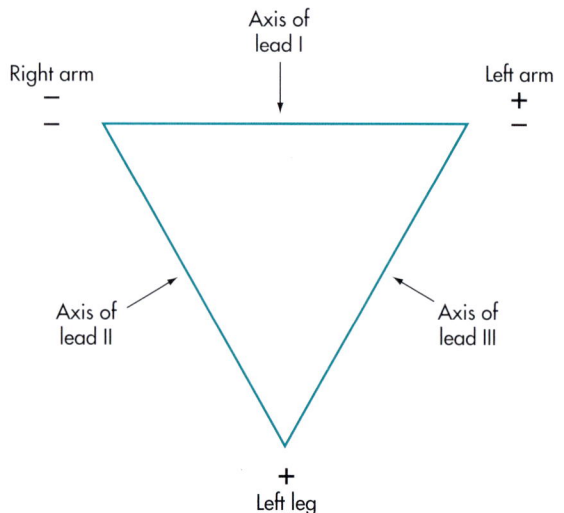

Figure 1.6 Einthoven's triangle

DETERMINING THE DIRECTION THE CURRENT IS TRAVELLING

- The current flowing towards a positive electrode is depicted by an upward deflection above the isoelectric line. Thus when the predominant portion of the wave complex is directed upward and above the isoelectric line, the current is travelling in that direction.

- The current flowing towards a negative electrode is depicted by a downward deflection below the isoelectric line. Thus when the predominant portion of the wave complex is directed downward and below the isoelectric line, the current is travelling away from that direction.

- The current flowing in a perpendicular direction to the positive and the negative electrodes will create a biphasic wave complex that has upward and downward deflections of equal size. Thus when the current is travelling in a neutral direction to two poles, the wave complex is bidirectional and balanced in size.

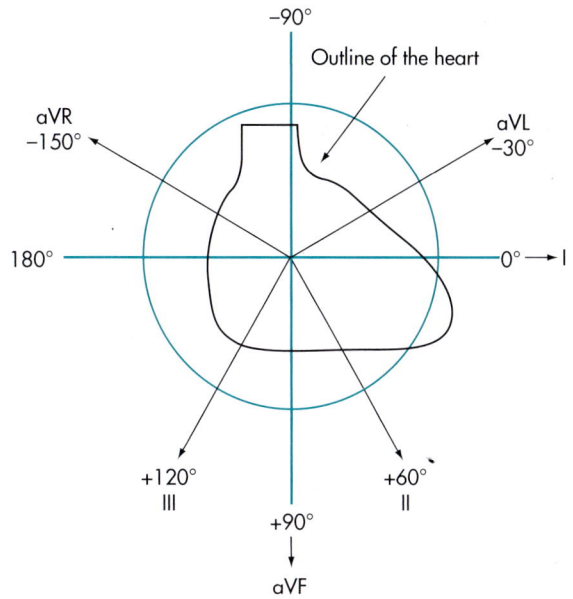

Figure 1.7 Hexa-axial reference system, also called the axis circle

DETERMINING THE CARDIAC AXIS

Determining the electrical axis in an ECG tracing is of fundamental importance. The axis indicates the direction along which the depolarisation wavefront in the heart (or the electrical current) is heading in the frontal plane of the human thorax. Normally, this axis is between −30° and +90° in the hexa-axial reference system shown in Figure 1.7. In other words, normally the current travels from the direction of the right shoulder to the direction of the left leg (from the top of the right atrium to the direction of the left ventricular apex).

Normally the average electrical current is directed towards the AV node, the point of entry of the depolarisation wavefront into the ventricles. Thus the usual direction of the current (also called the normal vector) is downwards and to the left; called the normal axis (Fig 1.8). When the axis is normal the QRS complex in the limb leads I and II will be predominantly upward, deflecting together with that of the augmented lead aVF.

The leftward direction of the current is depicted by the positive deflection in lead I, and the downward direction of the current by the positive deflection in lead aVF (Fig 1.9).

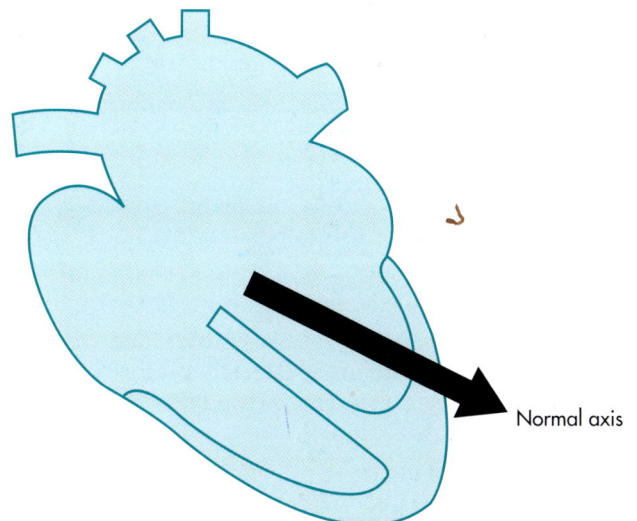

Figure 1.8 Cartoon of axis

METHODS TO DETERMINE THE CARDIAC AXIS

There are two rather simple methods to determine the cardiac axis, and the use of these is sufficient in most clinical situations. The first, the two-lead method, involves the observation of leads I and aVF, while the second, the three-lead method, involves leads I, II and III.

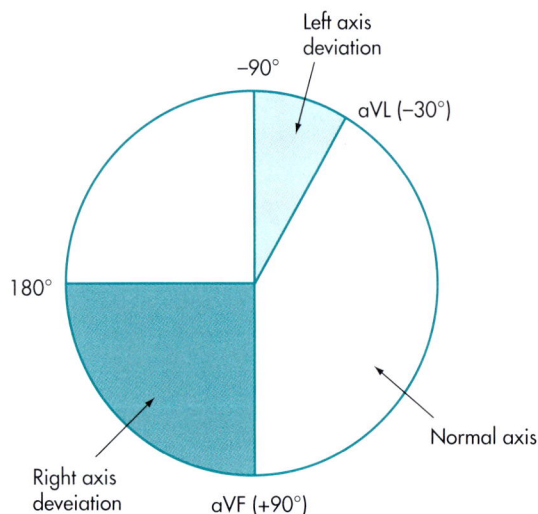

Figure 1.9 Normal axis (leads I, II and aVF)

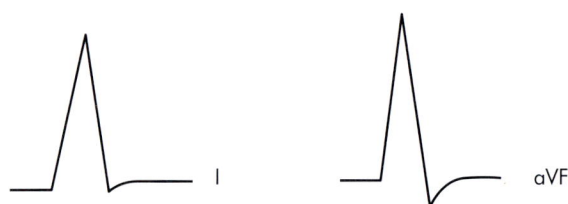

Figure 1.10 Normal axis, two-lead method

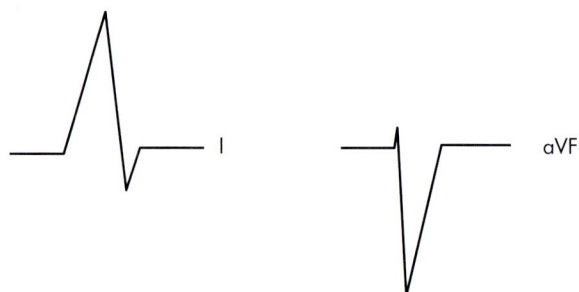

Figure 1.11 Left axis deviation, two-lead method

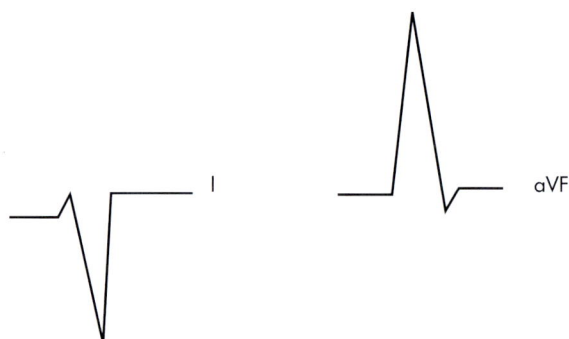

Figure 1.12 Right axis deviation, two-lead method

Two-lead method

NORMAL AXIS

Look at the QRS complexes in leads I and aVF. If both are predominantly positive (deflected above the isoelectric line), the axis is normal and the depolarising wavefront is directed towards the left lower quadrant between $-30°$ and $+90°$ in the circle (Fig 1.10).

LEFT AXIS DEVIATION

If the QRS complex in lead I is predominantly positive and that of lead aVF predominantly negative, the axis is directed to the left. Thus the direction of the depolarisation wavefront is to the left upper quadrant of the circle between $-30°$ and $-90°$ (left of $-30°$) (Fig 1.11).

RIGHT AXIS DEVIATION

If the QRS complex in lead I is predominantly negative and that of lead aVF is predominantly positive, the axis is directed to the right. The current is directed towards the right lower quadrant between $+90°$ and $+180°$ in the circle (right of $+90°$) (Fig 1.12).

Other possibilities for the axis

EXTREME RIGHT AXIS DEVIATION

If the QRS complexes of both lead I and aVF are deflected downward in the negative direction, the axis is called 'extreme'. In this case the depolarisation wavefront is directed towards the right upper quadrant between the angles of $+180°$ and $-90°$, and also called the 'Northwest territory' (the zone between the left axis and the right axis) (Fig 1.13). This is seen in ventricular tachycardia, right ventricular pacing and some cardiomyopathies.

UNDETERMINED AXIS

When the axis is directed in the transverse plane of the human thorax, that is, when it is perpendicular to the frontal plane, the axis is 'undetermined'. You will notice that all limb leads show iso-electricity or equal positive and negative deflections (Fig 1.14).

Figure 1.15 summarises the two-lead method.

Three-lead method

This method is based on determining the predominant direction of the three limb leads I, II and III.

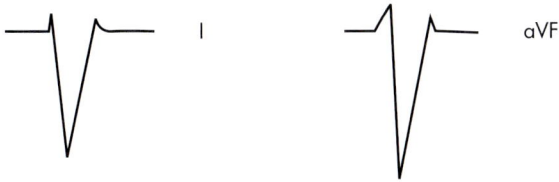

Figure 1.13 Extreme right axis deviation, two-lead method

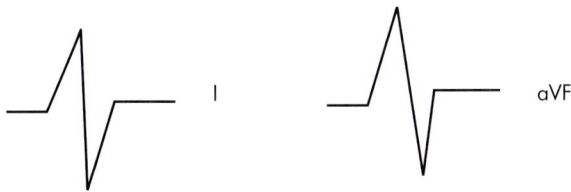

Figure 1.14 Undetermined axis, two-lead method

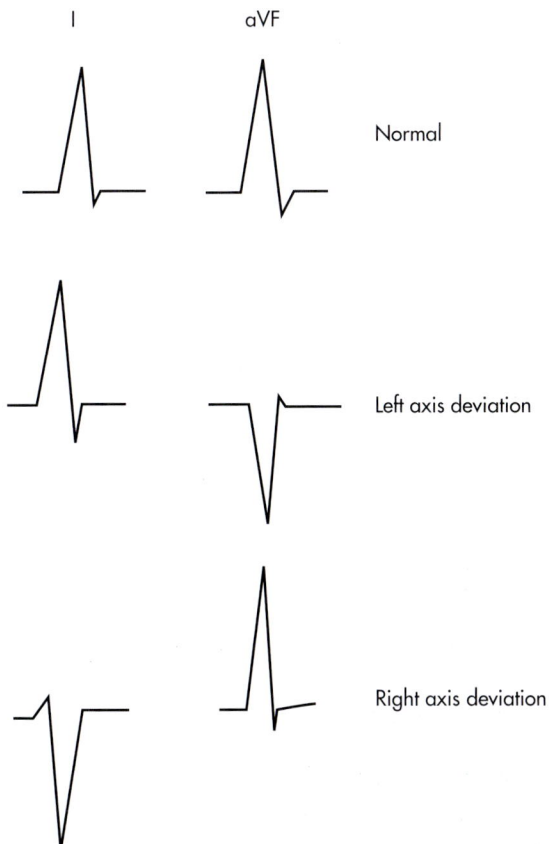

Figure 1.15 Summary of two-lead method

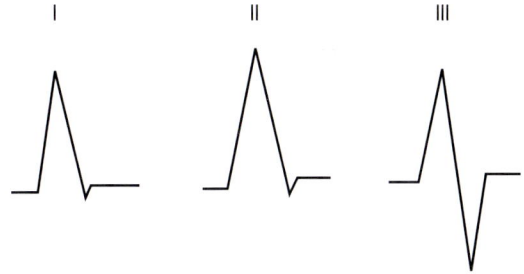

Figure 1.16 Normal axis, three-lead method

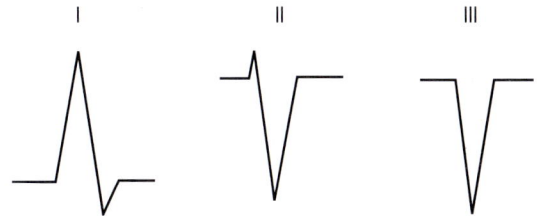

Figure 1.17 Left axis deviation, three-lead method

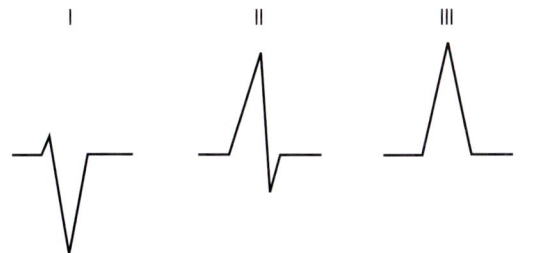

Figure 1.18 Right axis deviation, three-lead method

NORMAL AXIS
All three leads I, II and III show predominant upward deflections (Fig 1.16).

LEFT AXIS DEVIATION
If lead I shows predominantly upward deflection with leads II and III showing predominantly downward deflections, it is consistent with left axis deviation (Fig 1.17).

RIGHT AXIS DEVIATION
If lead I shows a predominantly downward deflection together with upward or biphasic deflection in lead II and predominantly upward deflection in lead III, it is consistent with right axis deviation (Fig 1.18).

EXTREME RIGHT AXIS DEVIATION
In this situation all three leads I, II and III show predominantly downward deflections.

THE MORE DIFFICULT, VERY ACCURATE METHOD

The most accurate technique involves understanding the position of each limb lead in the hexa-axial reference system. The first step is to look at the six limb leads (leads I, II, III, aVF, aVR, aVL) and identify the lead with the smallest QRS complex or the lead with equiphasic deflections (both deflections above and below the baseline of equal length) to determine the lead that has the most balanced biphasic waveform. Now refer to the hexa-axial reference system to find the lead that is perpendicular to the above lead. The direction of the current is along the axis of this lead. If this lead has a predominantly upward deflection, the current is directed towards the positive pole of this lead. If it has a predominantly downward deflection, the electrical axis is directed at the negative pole of this lead.

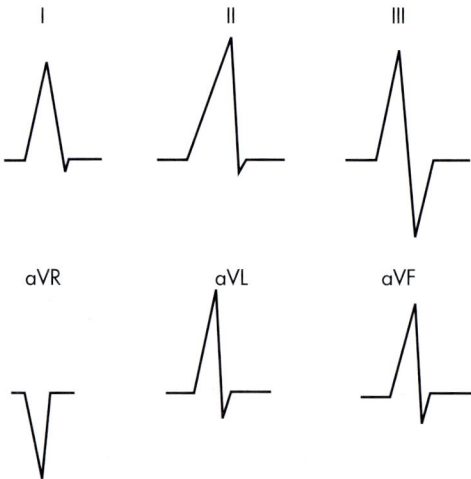

Note that in the hexa-axial reference system, each limb lead has a negative pole and a positive pole.

Figure 1.19 provides a step-by-step guide to accurate axis determination.

CAUSES OF LEFT AXIS DEVIATION

- Normal as a 'normal variation' or may be seen as an age-related change
- Pregnancy as the diaphragm is elevated
- Pathological causes of diaphragmatic elevation such as large ascites, and large abdominal masses or organomegaly
- Left ventricular hypertrophy
- Cardiac conduction defects, such as left bundle branch block or left anterior fascicular block
- Congenital heart defects, such as atrial septal defect (ASD)
- Pre-excitation or Wolff-Parkinson-White syndrome
- Ventricular tachycardia
- Hyperkalaemia
- Inferior myocardial infarction
- Emphysema
- Pacemaker-generated rhythm or paced rhythm

Step I: Note the equiphasic wave is in lead III

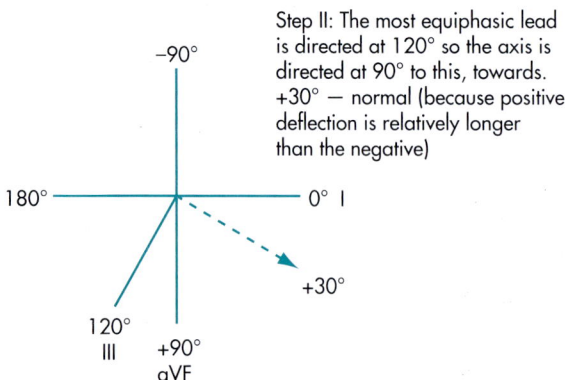

Step II: The most equiphasic lead is directed at 120° so the axis is directed at 90° to this, towards. +30° — normal (because positive deflection is relatively longer than the negative)

Figure 1.19 Guide to accurate axis determination

CAUSES OF RIGHT AXIS DEVIATION

- Normal variant just like left axis deviation, especially in children
- Pathological causes such as:
  » Right ventricular hypertrophy
  » Right bundle branch block
  » Left posterior fascicular block
  » Ventricular ectopic beats
  » Dextrocardia
  » Lateral wall infarction
- Conditions that can cause right ventricular strain such as pulmonary embolism, pulmonary hypertension, pulmonary stenosis, chronic lung disease and resultant cor pulmonale.

Note: In the setting of right bundle branch block, right or left axis deviation may indicate bifascicular block.

HOW TO PLACE THE ELECTRODES

ECG electrodes can detect cardiac electrical signals and generate a tracing. The leads are made up of negative and positive bipolar and unipolar electrodes. As discussed earlier, only the four limb electrodes are used to assess cardiac electrical activity from the surface of the body. Six different voltage measurements (or ECG tracings) were obtained from these four electrodes. However, a modern ECG recording involves six additional electrodes placed horizontally over the anterior aspect of the thorax. These are called chest electrodes; the voltage measured and recorded by these electrodes is represented by the six chest leads. To obtain a useful and accurate ECG tracing, the leads need to be placed at specific points on the body. The 12-lead ECG requires the placement of precordial or chest leads and limb leads. Body hair on hairy individuals may need to be shaved at the points where the electrodes are to be placed. Wipe away any sweat or other materials, such as lotions, to ensure the best contact with the skin. It is important to avoid bony prominences when placing electrodes.

Placement of leads on the thoracic region of the upper body should be done in the conventional manner so that the ECG recording can be properly interpreted. There are ten electrodes to be placed at predetermined positions, four limb electrodes and six chest electrodes, as discussed below.

Limb electrodes

The four limb electrodes need to be placed on the four limbs (Fig 1.20) as follows:

1   RA to be placed on the anterior surface of the right arm
2   LA to be placed on the anterior surface of the left arm (at the same level as the other arm electrode)
3   LL to be placed on the anterior aspect of the left leg
4   RL to be placed on the anterior aspect of the right leg (at the same level as the other leg electrode).

Usually the electrodes are marked according to where they should be placed, for example LL for left leg, LA for left arm.

Chest electrodes

Six chest electrodes need placement from the 4th intercostal space in the right margin of the sternum to the midaxillary line (Fig 1.20) as below:

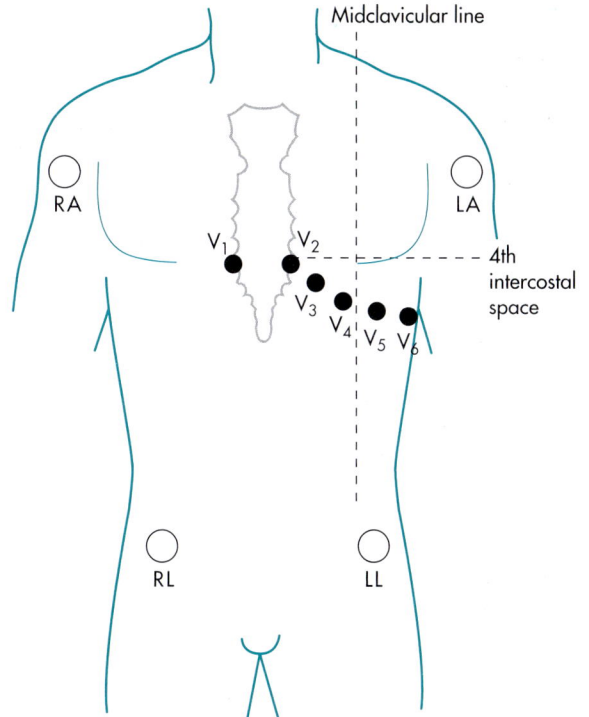

Figure 1.20 Electrode placement on the human body

1   V_1 to be placed on the 4th intercostal space directly next to the right margin of the sternum
2   V_2 to be placed on the 4th intercostal space directly next to the left margin of the sternum
3   V_3 to be placed directly between V_2 and V_4
4   V_4 to be placed on the 5th intercostal space on the left midclavicular line
5   V_5 to be placed horizontal to V_4, anterior on the left anterior axillary line
6   V_6 to be placed horizontal to V_4 and V_5 on the left midaxillary line.

Table 1.1 summarises the position of each electrode.

WHAT IS AN ELECTRODE AND WHAT IS A LEAD?

An electrode is a conductor through which electric current leaves the body. A lead is the electric potential (represented by the tracing) between two defined electrodes.

Figure 1.21 shows an ECG machine.

TABLE 1.1 Position of each electrode on the body	
Electrode label	**Position to be placed**
RA	On the right arm
LA	On the left arm
RL	On the right leg
LL	On the left leg
V_1	On the *fourth* intercostal space on the right sternal border
V_2	On the *fourth* intercostal space on the left sternal border
V_3	Between leads V_2 and V_4
V_4	On the fifth intercostal space on the midclavicular line
V_5	Horizontally at the same level as V_4 but on the anterior axillary line
V_6	Horizontally at the same level as V_4 and V_5 on the midaxillary line

ECG LEADS

The leads in the ECG denote voltage between electrodes placed according to the description above. The three types are limb leads, augmented limb leads and chest leads.

Limb leads

There are three limb leads I, II and III (Fig 1.22).

1 Lead I records the voltage between the left arm (LA) electrode, which is positive, and the right arm (RA) electrode, which is negative.

2 Lead II records the voltage between the left leg (LL) electrode, which is positive, and the right arm (RA) electrode, which is negative.

3 Lead III records the voltage between the left leg (LL) electrode, which is positive, and the left arm (LA) electrode, which is negative.

Augmented limb leads

There are three augmented limb leads, aVR, aVL and aVF, as shown in Figure 1.5. These leads are also derived from the same three limb electrodes I, II and III. However, they look at the heart from three different angles and thus read the electrical potential along these directions (Fig 1.23).

1 Lead aVR records the voltage between the right arm (RA) electrode, which is positive, and the combination of left arm (LA) and left leg (LL) electrodes that become the negative.

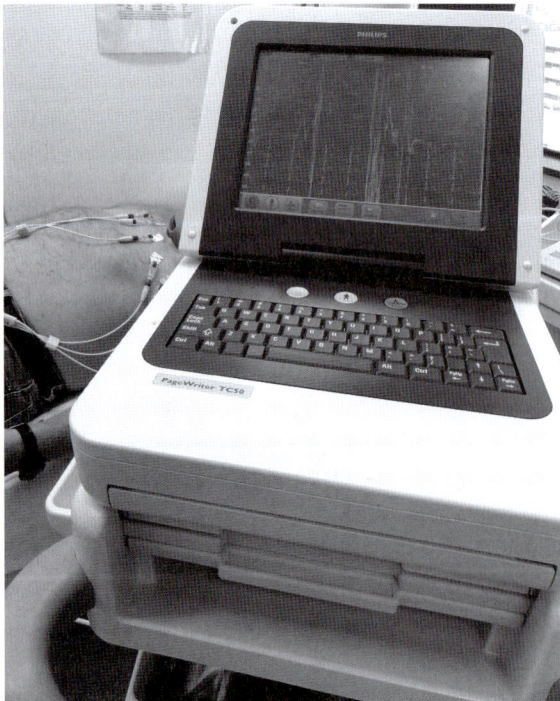

Figure 1.21 ECG machine

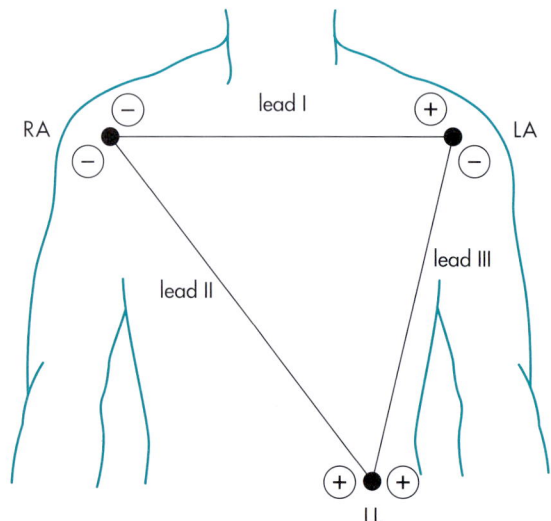

Figure 1.22 Limb leads

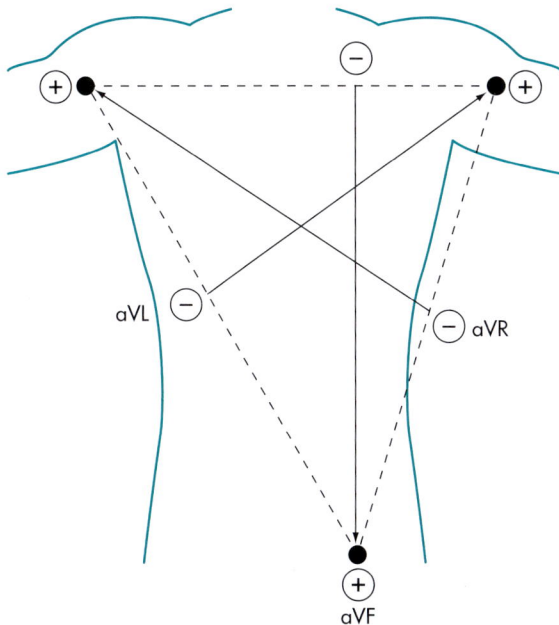

Figure 1.23 Augmented limb leads

This arrangement augments the electrical signal strength of the positive electrode RA.

2   Lead aVL records the voltage between the left arm (LA) electrode, which is positive, and the combination of right arm (RA) and left leg (LL) electrodes that become the negative. As before, this combination of negative electrodes augments the electrical signal strength of the positive electrode LA.

3   Lead aVF records the voltage between the left leg (LL) electrode, which is positive, and the combination of right arm (RA) and left arm (LA) electrodes that become the negative. Again, this combination of negative electrodes augments the electrical signal strength of the positive electrode LL.

Chest leads

There are six precordial or chest leads V_1, V_2, V_3, V_4, V_5 and V_6, as shown in Figure 1.24. The electrodes for these leads are placed on the chest wall along the precordium as described earlier.

These electrodes are unipolar and capable of recording the average potential at each particular point over the body. These leads describe the cardiac electrical activity in the horizontal plane. The heart's electrical axis in the horizontal plane is called the Z axis.

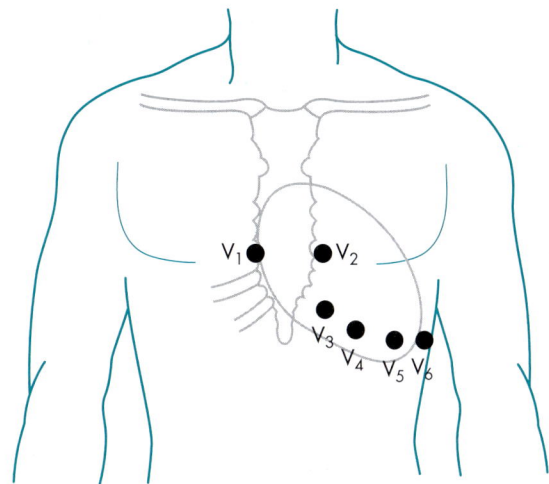

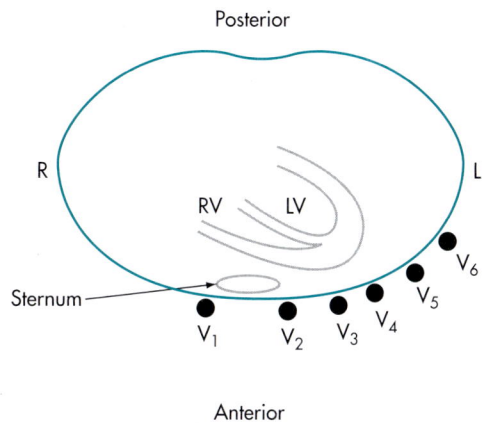

Figure 1.24 Chest leads

Note: Two ECG leads next to each other are called contiguous leads.

ECG LEADS AND CORRELATION TO REGION OF THE HEART

The ECG leads and correlations are shown in Figure 1.25.

- Lead I / Lead aVL / Lead V_5 / Lead V_6: examines the lateral aspect of the heart, mainly the lateral wall of the left ventricle.
- Lead II / Lead III / Lead aVF: examines the inferior aspect (diaphragmatic side) of the heart and the left ventricle.
- Lead V_1 / Lead V_2: examines the interventricular septum or the septal aspect of the heart.
- Lead V_3 / Lead V_4: examines the anterior aspect (or the sternocostal aspect) of the heart (left ventricle).

Right-sided ECG

As you can see, the standard 12-lead ECG described above detects predominantly the electrical activity of the left ventricle. To assess the possibility of the involvement of the right ventricle in an inferior wall myocardial infarction, a right-sided ECG needs to be obtained. This is done by placing precordial or chest leads across the right side of the body in a manner that is a mirror image of the left precordial lead placement (Fig 1.26), as follows:

- V_1R to be placed on the 4th intercostal space directly next to the left margin of the sternum
- V_2R to be placed on the 4th intercostal space directly next to the right margin of the sternum
- V_3R to be placed directly between V_2R and V_4R

- V_4R to be placed on the 5th intercostal space on the right midclavicular line
- V_5R to be placed horizontal to V_4R, anterior on the right anterior axillary line
- V_6R to be placed horizontal to V_4R and V_5R on the right midaxillary line.

Figure 1.27 shows a right-sided ECG.

Note that approximately half of inferior wall myocardial infarctions may have a right ventricular involvement. This is because in the majority of the population the inferior wall is supplied by the right coronary artery, which also gives away the

I lateral	aVR none	V_1 septal	V_4 anterior
II inferior	aVL lateral	V_2 septal	V_5 lateral
III inferior	aVF inferior	V_3 anterior	V_6 lateral

Figure 1.25 Leads and region of the heart

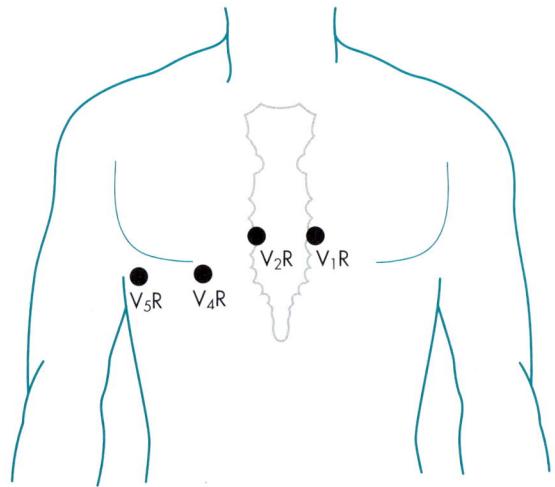

Figure 1.26 Electrode placement for right-sided ECG

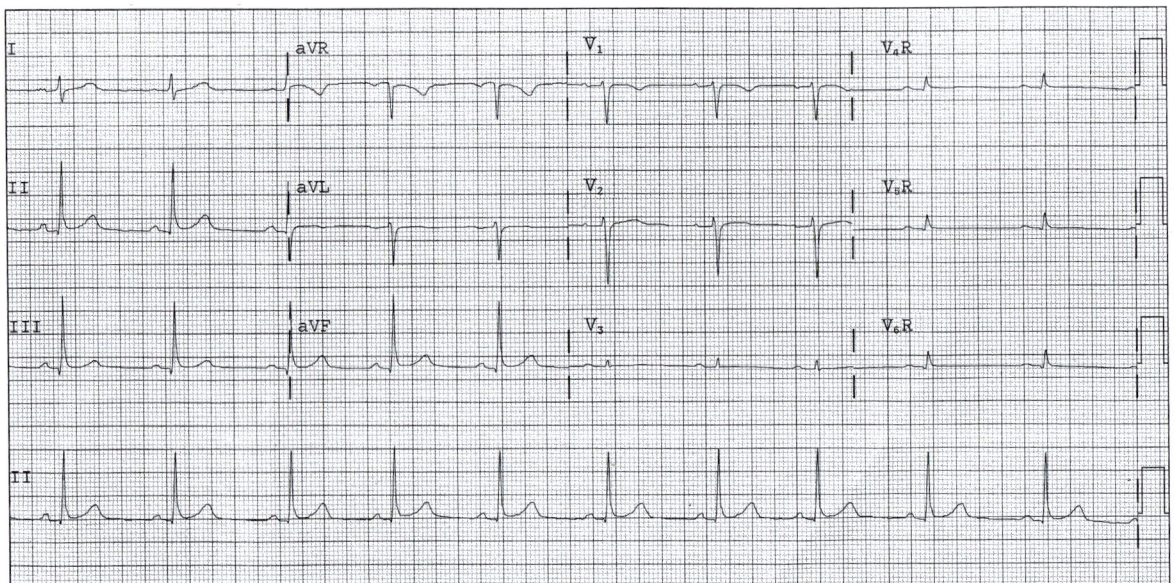

Figure 1.27 A right-sided ECG

right ventricular branch. If the occlusion is before the origin of the right ventricular branch, the right ventricle will suffer ischaemia.

Posterior ECG (and when it is indicated)

When there is a suspicion of a posterior wall myocardial infarction, it is important to place electrodes in the posterior aspect of the left thorax to record the electrical activity of the posterior aspect of the heart. Posterior leads are an extension of the precordial leads and include three additional leads V_7, V_8 and V_9. The placement of these leads, as shown in Figure 1.28, is:

- V_7 to be placed on the posterior axillary line on the 5th intercostal space (leadwire of V_4 is to be connected to this electrode)
- V_8 to be placed between V_7 and V_9 on the midscapular line at the same level (5th intercostal space) (leadwire of V_5 is to be connected to this electrode)
- V_9 to be placed just to the left of the spinal column (paraspinal line) on the 5th intercostal space (leadwire of V_6 is to be connected to this electrode)
- Recording will show activity only in the V_4, V_5 and V_6 leads on the ECG tracing that need to be relabelled as V_7, V_8 and V_9 respectively.

A posterior ECG with leads V_7, V_8 and V_9 is shown in Figure 1.29.

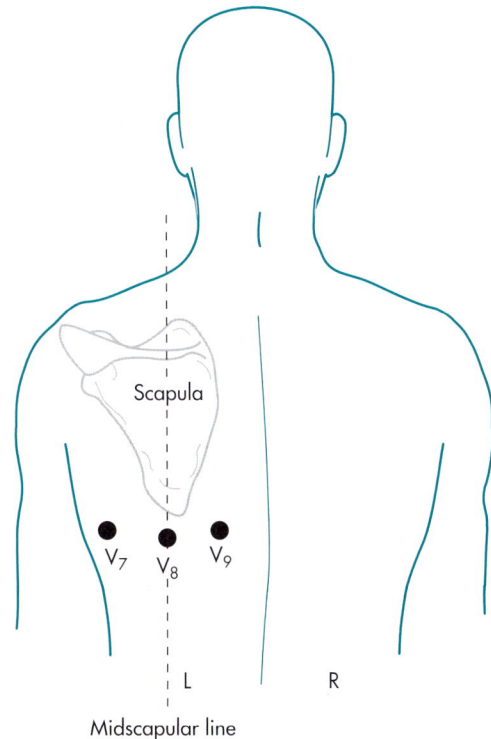

Figure 1.28 Electrode placement for posterior ECG

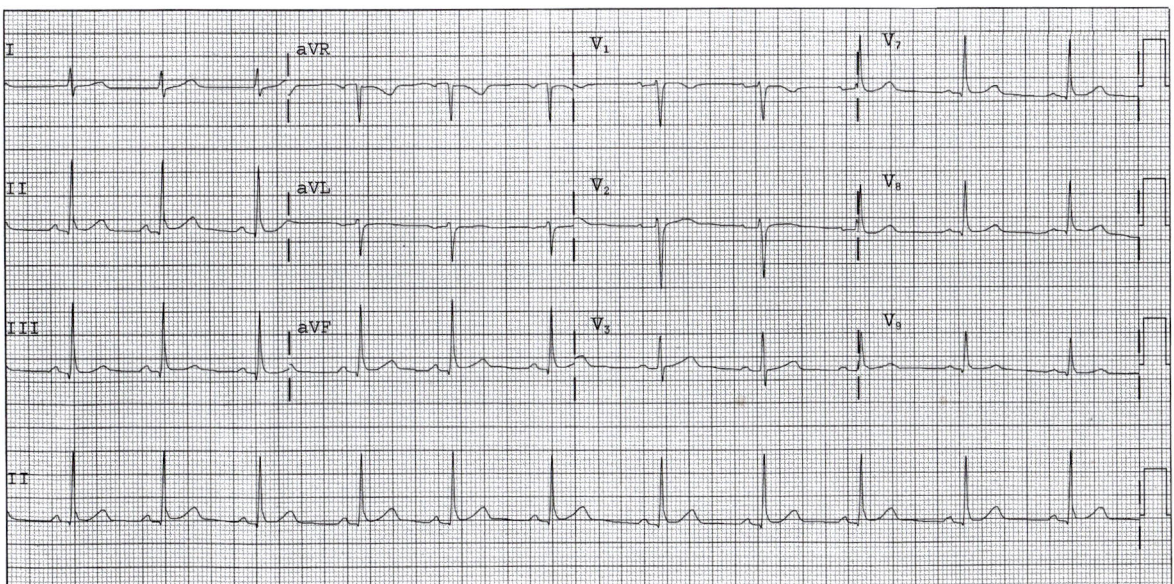

Figure 1.29 A posterior ECG with leads V_7, V_8 and V_9

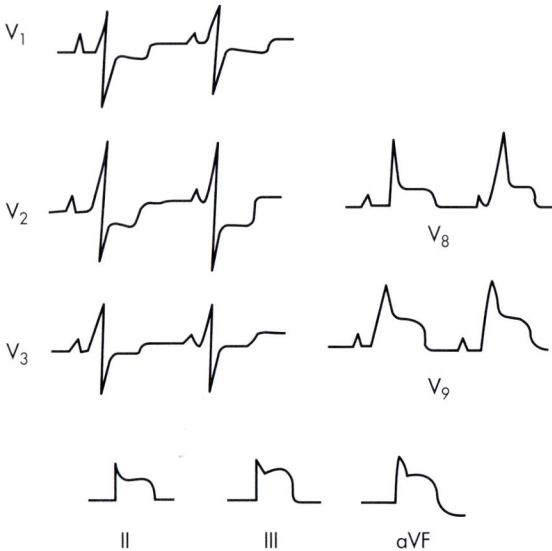

Figure 1.30 ECG changes that can indicate posterior wall infarction

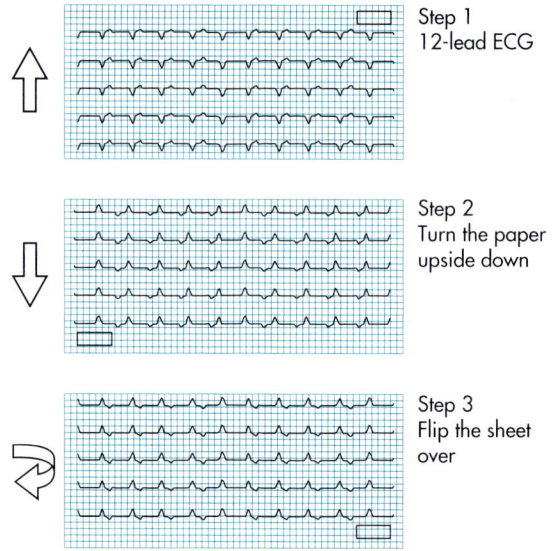

Step 1
12-lead ECG

Step 2
Turn the paper
upside down

Step 3
Flip the sheet
over

Changes of the standard left-sided ECG that suggest posterior wall infarction (Fig 1.30) are:

1   Tall R waves and ST segment depression in leads V_1 and V_2 (and sometimes in V_3, V_4 and even V_5)

2   You can perform 'mirror tests' of the above ECG by flipping the sheet over and turning it upside down (Fig 1.31). Look at it against a bright light and notice the changes of tall R waves appearing as Q waves, and the ST segment depressions as ST segment elevations!

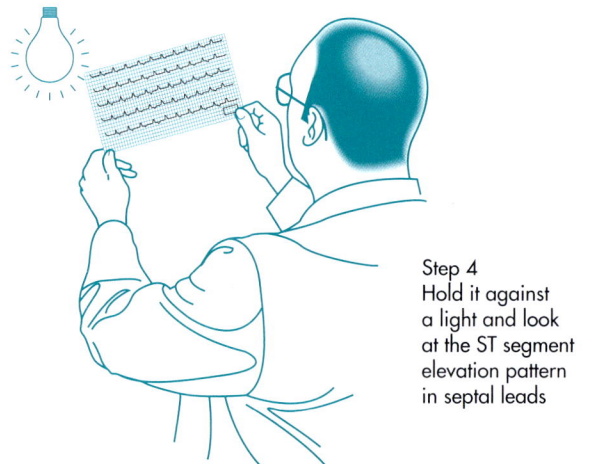

Step 4
Hold it against
a light and look
at the ST segment
elevation pattern
in septal leads

Figure 1.31 Guide to performing a mirror test

READING THE ECG

If you apply a standard practical algorithm for reading the ECG it is highly unlikely that you will miss any important and relevant information. Remember that we, as clinicians, treat the patient and not the ECG! Hence it is always important to correlate the ECG to the patient's clinical situation. Here we introduce a rather simple yet comprehensive framework for ECG interpretation. By using this framework every time you read an ECG, it will become habitual and practice will make it easy to use.

Practical rules for reading an ECG:

1   Identify the name of the patient

2   Check the date of birth of the patient

3   Identify the date the ECG was taken

4   Identify the scales used in the recording of the ECG (normal parameters are 1 millimetre per 1 millivolt and recording at a speed of 25 millimetres/second)

5   Look for obvious abnormalities that would warrant urgent action, such as ventricular tachycardia, ventricular fibrillation, severe bradycardia or ST elevation infarction

6   If the patient is stable, attempt interpreting the ECG in a systematic manner.

Systematic reading of the ECG

1 Establish the rate.
2 Establish the rhythm — regular or irregular (if irregular; *regularly* irregular or *irregularly* irregular)?
3 Establish the axis.
4 Identify the P wave — identify its morphology and size. If it is absent, think of atrial fibrillation or junctional rhythm.
5 Calculate the PR interval — normal PR interval is 200 milliseconds or less (5 small squares).
6 Look at the QRS complex — recognise the three waves. Observe the dimensions of the Q wave, R wave and S wave, their sizes and morphology. Check the length of the complex — is it wider than normal (more than 120 milliseconds or 3 small squares)? Is there a delta wave?
7 Identify the Q wave — significant if present and longer than one-quarter the length of the R wave.
8 Look at the ST segment — is it at the baseline, above it or below it? If displaced from the baseline, describe the morphology and dimensions (distance from the baseline).
9 Look at the T wave — is it upright, flat or inverted? Note its dimensions. Is it unusually tall?
10 Calculate the QT interval and correct it to the heart rate.
11 Check for the U wave.

THE NORMAL ECG

It is extremely important to familiarise yourself with the normal ECG (Fig 1.32). This mastery and familiarity with the normal ECG will enable you to identify abnormal or pathological ECGs quickly and more effectively (Table 1.2).

Sometimes the ECG of a healthy individual may have abnormal or pathological features. In the absence of symptoms or signs of the relevant pathology, these abnormalities are called normal variants. Thus it is very important to compare earlier ECGs to ascertain whether any changes seen in the current ECG are new or old. New ECG changes are important and often may suggest an underlying pathology.

Note the normal characteristics of the cardiac electrical complex:

- P wave — depicts the beginning of the depolarisation wave in the cardiac cycle. The vector of the current is from the SA node to the AV node or from the right atrium to the left atrium. Its duration is around 80 milliseconds (less than 120 milliseconds). The P wave is best observed in lead II. Its amplitude or height is less than 2.5 millimetres. Usually the P wave is upright but it could be biphasic in lead V_1.

- PR interval — depicts the conduction from the SA node to the ventricular tissue and the beginning of the QRS complex; normal duration is 150–200 milliseconds.

- QRS complex — depicts the depolarisation of the ventricles; normal duration is 80–120 milliseconds.

- ST segment — distance between the QRS complex and T wave; duration is 80–120 milliseconds.

- T wave — represents the repolarisation of the ventricle; the duration is 160 milliseconds. The height is less than 5 millimetres in the limb leads and less than 10 millimetres in the precordial leads.

- The distance between the beginning of the QRS complex and the apex of the T wave is the absolute refractory period of the ventricle. The segment from the apex of the T wave to its end

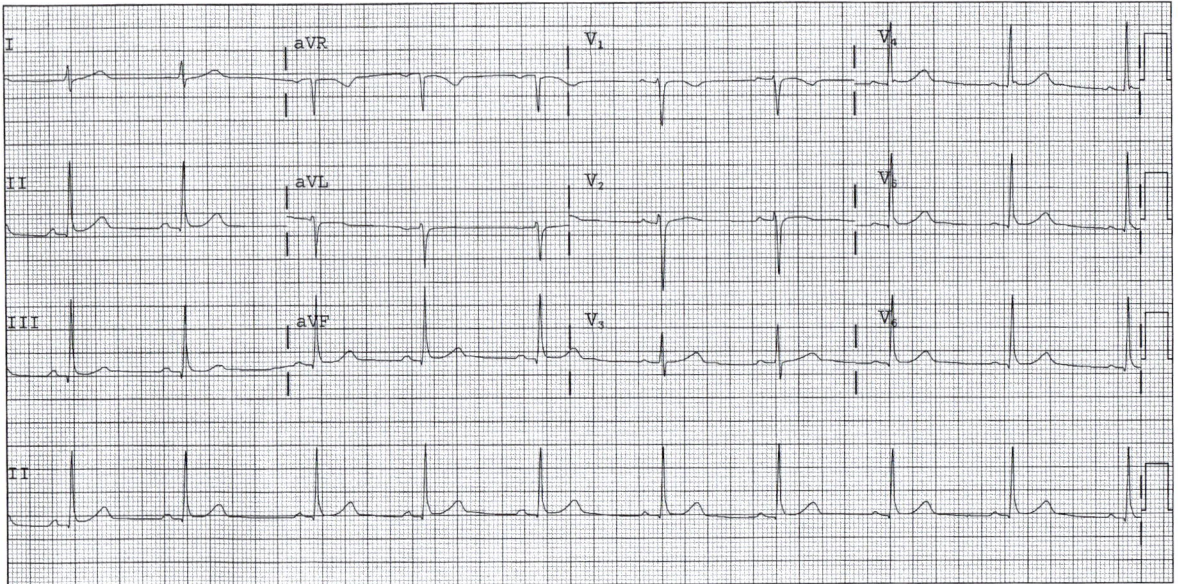

Figure 1.32 This normal ECG shows regular sinus rhythm at a rate of 60 beats per minute. The P wave, PR segment, QRS complex, ST segment and T wave all appear normal

TABLE 1.2 Normal ECG parameters		
Wave segment		**Length (ms)**
P wave	The impulse is generated in the SA node located in the right atrium. P wave highlights the migration of the impulse to the left atrium and the AV node.	80
PR segment	Section between the beginning of the P wave and the beginning of the R wave. It sits at the baseline.	150–200
QRS complex	Signifies the depolarisation of the ventricles. The point where the QRS complex ends and meets the ST segment is called the J (junctional) point.	80–120
ST segment	This segment is from the end of the S wave to the beginning of the T wave and sits on the isoelectric line. The ST interval by definition is from the J point of the QRS complex to the end of the T wave. Note this measurement is 300 ms.	80–120
T wave	The T wave represents the repolarisation phase of the ventricle.	160
QT interval	The QT interval is from the beginning of the QRS complex to the end of the T wave. This distance varies between males and females and also needs to be corrected to the heart rate. Once corrected for heart rate it is called the QTc interval.	350–450
U wave	Not always seen in the standard ECG. It is located just after the T wave and is usually of very low amplitude. It is considered to represent the repolarisation of papillary muscles.	

(second half of the T wave) represents the relative refractory period.

- QT interval — distance between the beginning of the QRS complex to the end of the T wave; normally it is 350–450 milliseconds. This interval incorporates both depolarisation and repolarisation of the ventricle. QT interval needs correction to the heart rate. The formula for the calculation of the corrected QT interval, called Bazzet's formula, is:

$$QTc = \frac{QT}{\sqrt{RR}}$$

where RR is the distance between two consecutive R waves measured in seconds (RR interval = 60/heart rate). Most computerised ECG machines automatically calculate this and state it in the interpretation.

- A QTc of more than 450 milliseconds in males and more than 470 milliseconds in females is abnormal and should be considered pathological.
- A U wave is usually very small and hence not seen. It can be upright or inverted, and it comes immediately after the T wave.

ECG-BASED DIAGNOSIS: PATHOLOGY BY ECG

ECG ABNORMALITIES

Abnormal electrocardiograms (ECGs) may provide valuable clues to an underlying pathology. The ECG should always complement a comprehensive clinical evaluation of the patient. The clinical evaluation consists of a thorough history, a detailed physical examination and the relevant bedside tests. Remember that we do not manage ECGs but patients!

To be able to spot abnormalities in ECGs it is extremely important first to be very familiar with the normal appearance of the 12-lead ECG, as shown in Figure 2.1. From a practical perspective, it is useful to organise ECG abnormalities and the underlying relevant pathologies in the same sequence used in Section 1 to read the ECG.

READING AN ECG: ITS RATE AND ABNORMALITIES

1. Abnormalities in the rate:
   - tachycardias or tachyarrhythmias — faster than normal rate (>100 bpm)
   - bradycardias or bradyarrhythmias — slower than normal rate (<50 bpm)
2. Abnormalities in the rhythm — regularly irregular or irregularly irregular
3. Abnormalities in the P wave
4. Abnormalities in the PR interval
5. Abnormalities in the QRS complex — broad complex with widening of the QRS complex, changes in the magnitude of the waveforms (height and depth)
6. Abnormalities in the ST segment
7. Abnormalities in the T wave in size or shape
8. Abnormalities in the QT interval
9. Appearance of a U wave
10. Appearance of a J or Osborn wave.

The normal rate at which heart muscle contracts is between 60 and 100 beats per minute (bpm).

TACHYCARDIA

Tachyarrhythmias

- Tachycardia is the rapid beating of the heart. A heart rate of over 100 bpm is considered tachycardia in adults. However in children the resting heart rate remains high, so in a child this definition would vary according to their age.
- Tachycardias are described according to the location of their origin since the pathological basis, management strategy and prognosis can be different.
- Tachycardias can be described as being narrow complex or broad complex. In narrow complex tachycardias, the QRS complex is equal to or shorter than 120 milliseconds (or 3 millimetre squares in width). In broad complex tachycardias this is longer than 120 ms or wider than 3 millimetre squares. Usually the supraventricular tachycardias (SVTs) are narrow complex unless there is an associated bundle branch block.
- The tachycardias can be divided into those that are supraventricular and those that are ventricular in origin, and can be described as regular or irregular.

Supraventricular tachycardia

This type of tachycardia is signified by a narrow QRS complex.

- SVTs can be of different types depending on their site of origin. The site of origin of an SVT has prognostic and management implications. Three types originate from the sinoatrial (SA) node, four types from atrial locations other than the SA node, and three types arise from around the junctional and atrioventricular (AV) node region.
- Some supraventricular tachycardias can be slowed down or terminated by vagal manoeuvres or drugs that suppress the AV node.

CLINICAL INFORMATION

The presenting symptoms of supraventricular tachycardia (SVT) are:

- Palpitation — described as the conscious (and often uncomfortable and anxiety provoking) feeling of one's heart beating fast
- Angina
- Dyspnoea
- Presyncope
- Syncope (usually rare with SVT)
- Stroke or transient ischaemic attacks (TIA) especially with atrial fibrillation

(a)

(b)

Device: Mobile 01   Speed: 25 mm/s   Limb: 10 mm/mV   Chest: 10 mm/mV

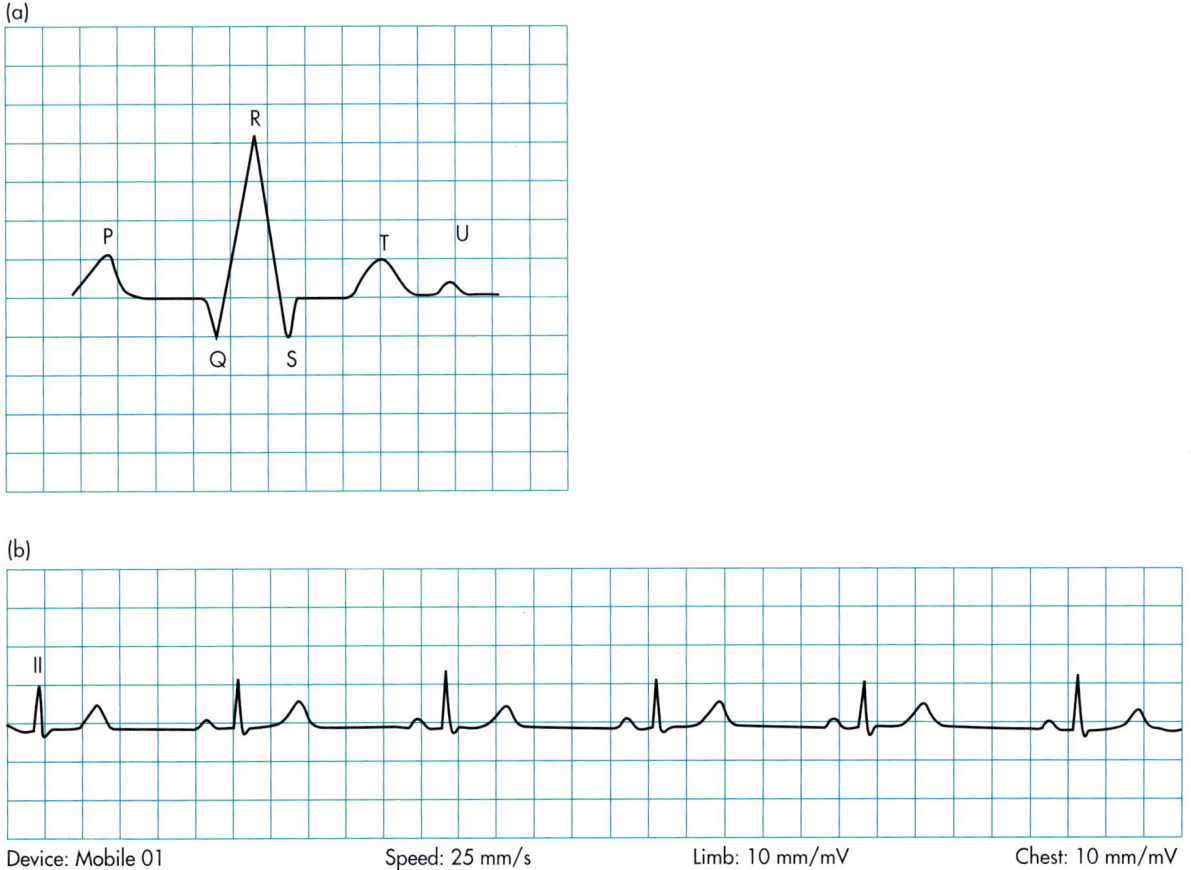

Figure 2.1 (a) Elements of the ECG complex; (b) normal rhythm and parameters

CLASSIFICATION OF SVTs BASED ON ORIGIN

SVTs originating from the SA node (three types)

- Sinus tachycardia — regular
- Inappropriate sinus tachycardia — regular
- Sinoatrial node reentrant tachycardia (SANRT) — regular

SVTs originating within the atria from a focus other than the SA node (four types)

- Multifocal atrial tachycardia (MAT) — irregularly irregular
- Focal atrial tachycardia (FAT) — regular >140 beats per minute
- Atrial fibrillation with a rapid ventricular rate — irregularly irregular
- Atrial flutter with a rapid ventricular rate — regular or irregular

SVTs originating from the junctional (AV) zone (three types)

- AV nodal reentrant tachycardia (AVNRT) — most common
- AV reentrant tachycardia (AVRT) — associated with an accessory AV conduction pathway and the second most common
- Junctional ectopic tachycardia (JET)

- Syndrome of heart failure including peripheral oedema, dyspnoea on exertion and at rest, orthopnoea and paroxysmal nocturnal dyspnoea. Heart failure can be caused by long-standing uncontrolled tachycardia, called tachycardia-induced cardiomyopathy.

Symptoms of SVT can occur as paroxysms at irregular intervals. Their onset and termination can be spontaneous, and their duration variable (a few minutes to hours or one to several days, or even until treated). If symptoms persist, medical intervention is required.

Tachycardia can cause hypotension due to inadequate filling of the left heart during diastole because of the reduced filling time. It can also cause angina due to inadequate filling of the coronaries during diastole, particularly in those patients with coronary artery disease.

DETAILED EXPLANATION OF SVT TYPES

The individual subtypes of SVT can be distinguished from each other by certain physiological and electrical characteristics. Many of these features are represented in the patient's ECG.

SVTs originating from the SA node

Sinus tachycardia

The rate is over 100 bpm. The duration of the QRS complex is normal and each QRS complex is preceded by a P wave. Sinus tachycardia is a normal response to stress. Stressors include physical exercise, hypovolaemia, dehydration, emotional excitement (such as fright), severe anaemia, sepsis, fever, catecholamine surge and adrenergic medications (such as beta agonists given as bronchodilators).

Inappropriate sinus tachycardia

This is similar to sinus tachycardia but persists without any clear trigger factor or stimulus; hence the term inappropriate. Its aetiology is not clear. It responds to pharmacotherapeutics such as beta-blockers and ivabradine. Resistant cases may require electrophysiological study and radiofrequency ablation.

Sinoatrial node reentrant tachycardia (SANRT)

In this rhythm the P wave is of normal character and it precedes each QRS complex. The QRS complex is narrow and of normal duration. In its features it is identical to sinus tachycardia. However unlike sinus tachycardia, it is not due to any physical stimuli or stressors as its onset is spontaneous. It can self terminate or require treatment for termination. It responds well to vagal manoeuvres, unlike sinus tachycardia that persists till the stimulus is removed. SANRT is caused by a reentry circuit within the SA node.

SVTs originating within the atria from a focus other than the SA node

Multifocal atrial tachycardia (MAT)

This rhythm can be irregular with narrow QRS complexes that are preceded by P waves. The P waves are of different morphologies (usually three or more) varying in shape and size, but a P wave is always present before each QRS complex. It is seen in the elderly and is associated with lung disease or heart failure. This rhythm eventually degenerates into atrial fibrillation (AF).

Focal atrial tachycardia (FAT)

In this rhythm each QRS complex is preceded by an abnormal-looking P wave. It is a regular rhythm that originates from a single localised ectopic focus in the left or right atrium and it overrides sinus rhythm. Its rate can vary between 120–300 bpm.

Atrial fibrillation with a rapid ventricular rate

The rhythm here is irregularly irregular (Fig 2.4). There are no discrete P waves but irregular fibrillatory waves interspersed between QRS complexes. Ventricular response could be rapid (causing tachycardia) or controlled at a rate of below 100 bpm.

Atrial flutter

In this rhythm the flutter waves or F waves appear as 'saw-tooth' shaped waveforms (Fig 2.5). These are best seen in lead II, usually at a rate of 300 bpm, and are regular. Depending on the degree of block at the level of the AV node, the ventricular response could be 300, 150 or 75 bpm.

> **Degree of block** defines how many atrial beats are allowed into the ventricle by the AV node. If all beats are allowed in it is called one to one conduction. If every second beat is allowed in it is called two to one block. If every third beat is allowed in it is called three to one block.

If the ventricular rate is 300 bpm, then there is one to one conduction. If it is 150 bpm (it can vary between 130 and 150), then there is an AV nodal block of two to one. If the rate is 100 bpm, the block is three to one. Usually the rhythm is regular, however if there is a variable AV block the ventricular response can be irregular but in between QRS complexes you can see regular flutter waves.

Usually the cause of atrial flutter is a reentry circuit around the tricuspid valve annulus that can be interrupted by radiofrequency ablation, thus curing the arrhythmia.

SVTs originating from the junctional (AV) zone

AV nodal reentrant tachycardia (AVNRT) [also called junctional reciprocating tachycardia]

This is the most prevalent type of SVT (Fig 2.2). The QRS complexes are narrow and regular. You may see a retrograded conducted P wave buried within the QRS complex or occurring just after the QRS complex.

This tachyarrhythmia is due to a reentry circuit situated just adjacent to the AV node or within the AV node. Both pathways are located in the right atrium. The two pathways involved in the reentry circuit have different speeds of impulse conduction: one is a fast conducting pathway and the other a slow pathway. In the more common variety, antegrade conduction is via the slow pathway and retrograde conduction is via the fast pathway.

The condition is more common among females (75% of the presentations). It can be controlled by oral AV node blocking agents, such as beta-blockers, verapamil or diltiazem. Those who are intolerant or resistant to medical therapy need referral for electrophysiological study and radiofrequency ablation of the abnormal pathway. During ablation the slow pathway, which is located inferior and posterior (near the origin of the coronary sinus) to the SA node, is burnt with radiofrequency energy. The fast pathway is located superior and posterior to the SA node.

Atrioventricular reentrant tachycardia (AVRT) [also known as circus movement tachycardia (CMT)]

This is the second most common type of SVT (Fig 2.3). It is a narrow (or rarely, broad when there is a block or a delta wave) complex tachycardia with

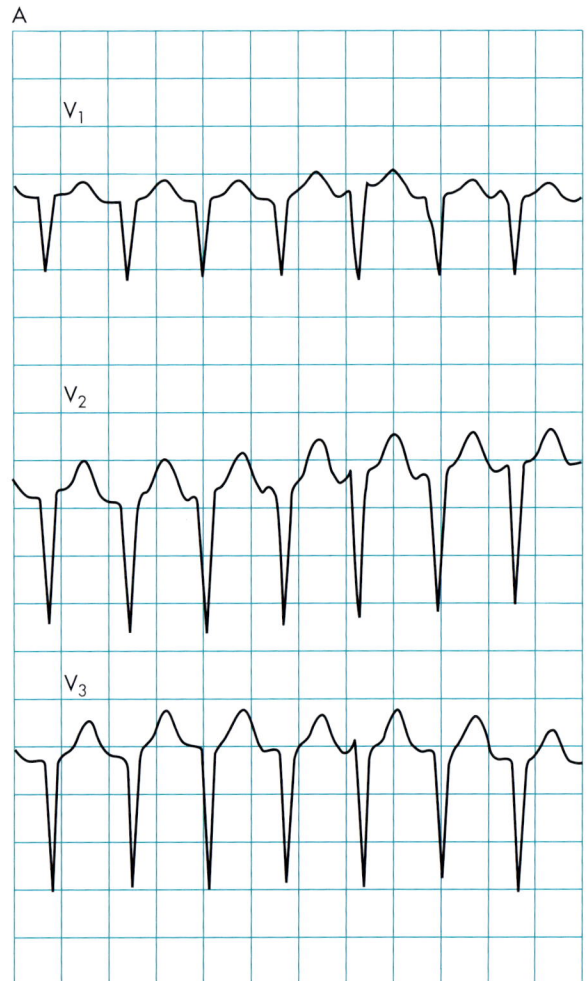

Figure 2.2 AV nodal reentrant tachycardia

a short PR interval. An accessory pathway connects the atria to the ventricles. The tachycardia is due to the reentry of impulses from the ventricles back to the atria, creating a self-sustained circuit. One arm of the reentry circuit is formed by the accessory pathway and the other by the usual AV nodal pathway. Because the accessory pathway is located away from the AV node, the reentry circuit is larger than in AVNRT.

If the accessory pathway conducts the atrial impulse to the ventricle, a slurred upstroke will be seen at the beginning of the QRS complex. This is called the delta wave.

The two types of AVRT are:

1 Orthodromic AVRT

The P wave occurs after each narrow QRS complex. The antegrade (atrium to ventricle)

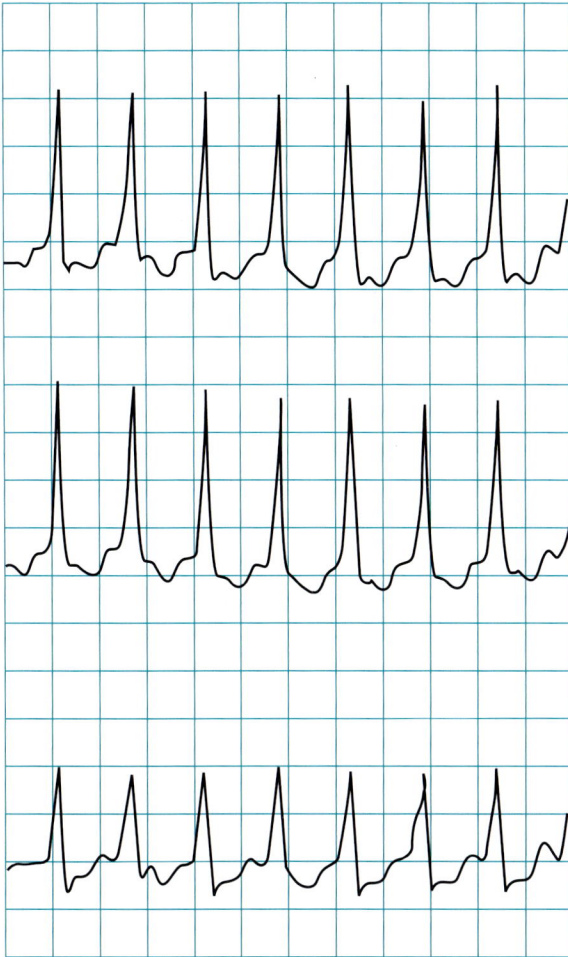

Figure 2.3 AVRT: note the delta value on the QRS complex, the P wave that precedes the QRS complex and the short PR interval—this is antidromic AVRT

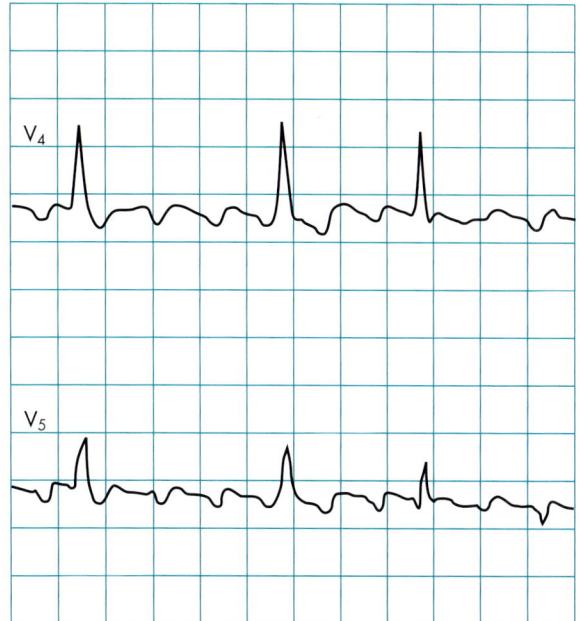

Figure 2.4 Atrial fibrillation: note the irregularly irregular tachycardia

conduction of the atrial impulse is via the AV node. The impulse is then conducted back (retrograded) to the atrium via the accessory pathway. This is called orthodromic AV reentrant tachycardia. Since the accessory pathway is not conducting antegradely, it is called a concealed accessory pathway (no delta wave is seen in the ECG).

2 Antidromic AVRT

The P wave occurs before the QRS complex with a very short PR interval. The antegrade conduction is via the accessory pathway that has a shorter refractory period and a faster conduction speed. The antegrade conduction via the accessory pathway causes the broadening of

the QRS complex by creating a delta wave that appears as a slurred upstroke as described above. Reentry of the impulse back to the atria happens via the AV node thus completing the reentry circuit.

Junctional ectopic tachycardia (JET)

This tachycardia originates at the atrioventricular junction in the AV node. It is a narrow QRS complex tachycardia with P waves that can be seen at different locations with no clear relationship to the QRS complexes. QRS complexes occur at regular intervals. Some P waves are retrogradely conducted. These P waves may appear inverted. This tachycardia is caused by increased abnormal automaticity of the AV node. This is very rare and is often related to medication toxicity.

MANAGEMENT

Immediate termination or slowing of the rhythm is indicated if the patient is symptomatic. Most SVTs that require AV nodal conduction for propagation may slow down or even terminate with vagal manoeuvres that cause inhibition of the AV nodal conduction. Management options for SVTs are as follows.

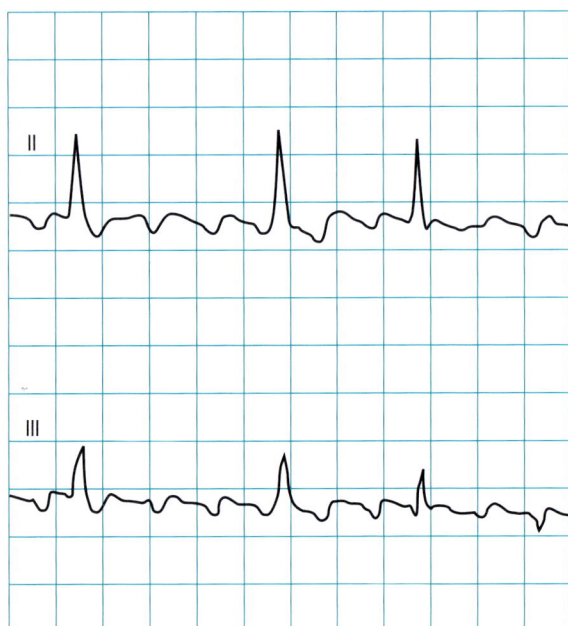

Figure 2.5 Atrial flutter: note the saw-tooth shaped flutter waves

DC shock or electrical cardioversion

This is required when there is haemodynamic instability or severe symptoms due to the tachyarrhythmia. It is also indicated when all other measures have failed. Rapid reversion to sinus rhythm can be achieved by DC electrical cardioversion. DC shock therapy should not be given in digoxin toxicity, sinus tachycardia or multifocal atrial tachycardia. Adequate therapeutic anticoagulation is required before and after DC cardioversion of AF.

Vagal manoeuvres

Carotid sinus massage

Apply gentle but firm pressure on the carotid body located at the midpoint between the angle of the mandible and the superior border of the thyroid cartilage. Start with the right side and continue massaging for 5 seconds at a time with concurrent ECG monitoring. Do not perform carotid sinus massage if there is carotid bruit. A carotid bruit may be due to an underlying carotid plaque that could rupture if the artery is massaged.

Valsalva manoeuvre

Perform this manoeuvre by forcibly exhaling against a closed glottis (with both the nose and the mouth sealed). Monitor the patient's ECG in real time.

Other methods to increase vagal tone

- Holding breath for a short period
- Dipping face in cold water
- Sipping ice cold water.

AV node blocking agents

- **Adenosine** can be given at a dose of 6 mg as an intravenous push followed by further 12 mg given after 1–2 minutes if required. Concurrently monitor the ECG. Adenosine has a very short half-life. Adenosine is usually not used in rapid AF where a more sustained effect is required.
- **Verapamil** can be given at a dose of 5–10 mg as a slow IV push over 3 min.
- **Diltiazem** can be given at a dose of 0.25 mg/kg over 2 min as an IV push.

  Other agents that block the AV node include beta-blockers, digoxin and diltiazem.
- **Beta-blockers,** such as atenolol, can also be given in this situation. Atenolol is administered at a dose of 1–3 mg as an IV push, slowly over 4 min.

  Digoxin is less potent in this situation. It is given at a loading dose of 0.5–1 mg infusion over 2 hours. The maintenance dose could be 62.5–250 mcg daily.

  All of the above drugs can be given orally for long-term control of SVT.

Other anti-arrhythmic drugs

Sotalol, amiodarone or flecainide can be given but only when there is no structural heart disease.

Long-term management

Long-term management goals include prevention and cure. Prevention of recurrent episodes can be achieved with the following agents given orally on a regular basis:

- AV node blocking agents, such as beta-blockers, calcium channel blockers and digoxin. AV nodal blocking agents should not be given if there is evidence of Wolff-Parkinson-White syndrome.
- Class Ic and III anti-arrhythmic agents — flecainide (belongs to Class Ic) and sotalol, ibutilide, amiodarone, dronedarone (belong to Class III). Amiodarone is less preferred in this context due to its side effect profile. Ibutilide is

used to treat AF and atrial flutter. Dronedarone is used to treat atrial fibrillation.

- For those with Wolff-Parkinson-White syndrome — flecainide (Class I) or sotalol (Class III). AV nodal blocking agents could cause VF in patients with Wolff-Parkinson-White syndrome and hence it is contraindicated.

Radiofrequency ablation — This is curative in most cases. Indications include recurrent episodes despite drug therapy, symptomatic Wolff-Parkinson-White syndrome and significant adverse impact on quality of life. Selected cases of AF can be treated with radiofrequency ablation of the pulmonary venous ostia (pulmonary venous isolation).

CLINICAL NOTES ON AF

AF is the most common arrhythmia. It is more common among older people and the elderly. The causative associations of AF include: ischaemic heart disease, chronic hypertension, diabetes, heart failure, mitral or tricuspid valve disease, thyroid disease, family history and alcohol excess.

Patients with AF present with palpitation, angina, dyspnoea and presyncope. Diagnosis is made by the detection of an irregularly irregular pulse and confirmed by ECG. Echocardiogram is a useful investigation in this setting.

Management of AF involves rate control, rhythm control and stroke prevention. Rate control is achieved by drugs that block the AV node, such as beta-blockers, non-dihydropyridine calcium channel blockers and digoxin.

Rhythm control can be achieved by DC cardioversion or anti-arrhythmic agents, such as amiodarone, dronedarone, sotalol, flecainide and ibutilide. A select group of patients may be effectively treated with radiofrequency ablation of the ostia of the pulmonary veins in the left atrium. The need for rate control or rhythm control is based on the patient's symptoms, tolerance to medication and age. Evidence dictates that neither strategy is superior to the other.

AF significantly increases the risk of thromboembolic stroke. Additional risk factors can increase this risk. Risk of AF is similar for intermittent AF and chronic AF. This risk can be measured by the CHADS2 score: patients who score more than 1 need therapy for stroke prevention.

CHADS2 score algorithm

- Cardiac failure — 1 point
- Hypertension — 1 point
- Age ≥ 75 years — 1 point
- Diabetes — 1 point
- Stroke or TIA history — 2 points.

Those who score 0 are at lower risk of stroke. Those who score 1 may benefit from aspirin, warfarin or dabigatran. Those who score ≥ 2 benefit from warfarin or dabigatran therapy.

A patient with AF due to valvular heart disease will benefit from anticoagulation no matter what their CHADS2 score is. Those who do not tolerate anticoagulation may benefit from the occlusion of the left atrial appendage with the Plato device that can be delivered percutaneously.

PRACTICAL NOTES ON DC CARDIOVERSION

1 Patient needs to be given general anaesthesia or conscious sedation.
2 Place the pads on patient's thorax.
3 Set the dial to select the shock energy and press the charge button.
4 The first shock can be given at 100–200 J; if that fails give further shocks at 360 J. Biphasic devices need only lower energy shocks initially and for AF the first shock can be at 75 J.
5 Press the 'synch' button to synchronise to the patient's heartbeat.
6 Press the shock button when charged, ready and safe.
7 Check the ECG monitor for the result.

VENTRICULAR TACHYCARDIA

These are tachycardias that originate from a focus in the ventricles. They are characterised by a broad QRS complex (larger than 120 ms). Based on the morphology, VT is classified as polymorphic or monomorphic. In monomorphic VT all QRS complexes look alike. Polymorphic VT is also called torsades de pointes.

If the VT duration is more than 30 s, it is considered to be sustained VT.

VT can cause haemodynamic collapse and degenerate into ventricular fibrillation (VF) leading to sudden cardiac death or cardiac arrest. So, due to the high risk of clinical urgency associated with VT, all broad complex tachycardias should be considered as VT until proven otherwise.

The other differential diagnosis of VT is SVT with aberrancy or bundle branch block, or SVT with a delta wave as in Wolff-Parkinson-White syndrome.

The different types of wide complex tachycardia

1   Ventricular tachycardia (most common and seen in over 80 per cent of cases)
2   SVT with aberrancy (due to a conduction delay or bundle branch block)
3   Tachycardia with pre-excitation (such as Wolff-Parkinson-White syndrome)
4   Tachycardia with paced rhythm.

R on T phenomenon

If an ectopic beat falls on the down sloping segment of the T wave, this can trigger ventricular tachycardia. This is called the R on T phenomenon, and is often observed at the transition from sinus rhythm to VT on an ECG strip.

ECG features to note in VT

The rate is more than 100 bpm. The QRS complex is wide (usually over 140 ms). There is evidence of dissociation between the impulses generated in the atrium and ventricle (this phenomenon is called AV dissociation). All QRS complexes in the chest leads show either positive or negative deflection. This phenomenon, called QRS *concordance in the chest leads*, is a distinguishing feature of VT.

FEATURES OF AV DISSOCIATION

1   QRS complexes that are independent of P waves. There may be occasional P waves scattered between the wide QRS complexes with no real association to them, so the P waves bear no relationship to the QRS complexes that originate from the ventricle.
2   Capture beats (escape beats). There may be occasional narrow QRS complexes embedded between wide complexes, each preceded by an identifiable P wave. These sinus beats that escape into the ventricle are called 'capture beats'.

3   Fusion beats. Some beats show features of sinus complexes fused with a ventricular complex; they are called 'fusion beats'.

There are also subtle differences in the QRS complexes, which is called beat-to-beat variation.

Note that VT with a left bundle branch block (LBBB) pattern originates in the right ventricle and that a right bundle branch block (RBBB) pattern originates in the left ventricle.

DIAGNOSTIC CRITERIA FOR VT

Electrophysiologists have attempted to define diagnostic ECG criteria for VT. There are four sets of criteria most commonly used in practice. These include Brugada criteria, AHA criteria, Wellens criteria and Josephson criteria, as discussed below. Of these, Wellens criteria are for the diagnosis of VT with a RBBB morphology and Josephson criteria are for the diagnosis of VT with a LBBB morphology.

Brugada criteria for wide complex tachycardia with LBBB or RBBB pattern[1]

In 1991 two Spanish electrophysiologists named Brugada (they are brothers) published a list of criteria based on observations made from analysing over 500 ECGs with wide complex tachycardia. They incorporated these criteria into an algorithm of inclusions as given below.

Step 1: Look for any RS complexes in the precordial or chest leads. If no precordial lead shows an RS complex it is VT. *If this criterion is not fulfilled go to Step 2.*

Step 2: Measure the R to S interval (distance from the beginning of the R wave to the nadir of the S wave) in the precordial leads (where RS complex is present). If any one complex has an R to S interval of more than 100 ms, it is VT. See the R to S interval in Figure 2.6. *If this criterion is not met go to Step 3.*

Step 3: Look for AV dissociation: if present it is VT. *If absent go to Step 4.*

Step 4: Look at the precordial leads and decide whether it shows LBBB pattern or RBBB pattern.

» If it is LBBB pattern, see whether V_1 has the following features: R wave of >30 ms, distance to S wave nadir >60 ms, a notch in the S wave. Now look at V_6 for a Q wave. These features suggest VT.

» If it is RBBB pattern, look at V_1 for a monophasic complex or a QR or RS pattern.

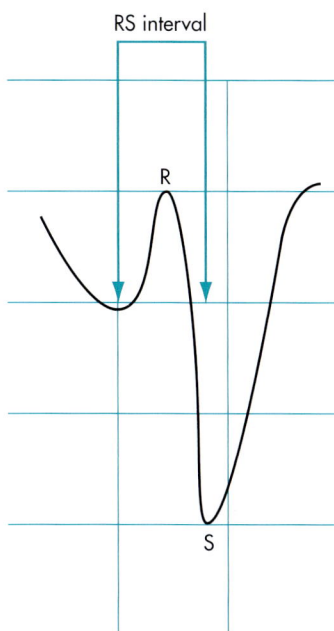

Figure 2.6 The RS interval

Then look at V_6 for a smaller R wave when compared to the S wave, a QR or QS complex, or a monophasic R wave: these features indicate VT. (A triphasic QRS complex in V_1 or V_6 is suggestive of SVT with aberrancy.)

AHA criteria for the diagnosis of VT

The American Heart Association (AHA) has published the following broad criteria for the diagnosis of VT:

1 Atrioventricular dissociation
2 QRS axis between $-90°$ and $\pm180°$
3 Positive QRS concordance (positive QRS V_1–V_6)
4 QRS duration of 140 ms or more with RBBB pattern and 160 ms or more with LBBB pattern
5 Combination of LBBB pattern and right axis
6 Monophasic or biphasic QRS complex with RBBB pattern and slurred or prolonged S wave in V_1 with LBBB morphology.

Wellens criteria for wide complex tachycardia (with RBBB pattern)[2]

The presence of the following features favours the diagnosis of VT:

1 QRS complex duration of more than 140 ms
2 Left axis deviation

3 AV dissociation
4 Capture and/or fusion beats
5 RSR pattern in V_1, mono or biphasic QRS in V_1, or monophasic QS in V_6.

Josephson criteria for VT (with LBBB morphology)[3]

1 Presence of a small notch in the S wave close to its nadir indicates VT
2 R wave in V_1 or V_2 of more than 40 ms
3 Duration from the onset of QRS complex to the nadir of S wave more than 60 ms in V_1 and V_2
4 Any Q wave in V_6.

HOW TO DIFFERENTIATE BETWEEN VT AND SVT WITH ABERRANCY

SVT with aberrancy will give a broad complex tachycardia on ECG due to LBBB or RBBB. This may look like VT, hence it is important to distinguish between the two in the haemodynamically stable patient. The management is different and the prognosis is worse with VT. Important points to remember in this setting include:

1 VT is the most common wide complex tachycardia, so it is more common than SVT with aberrancy
2 If the patient has predisposing factors, such as ischaemic heart disease, heart failure, cardiomyopathy and so on, it is more likely to be VT
3 In those who are over the age of 35 years, VT is more common
4 Axis deviation to the extreme right (northwest) ($-90°$ to $\pm180°$) is suggestive of VT
5 A negative QRS complex in V_1 together with right axis deviation is suggestive of VT
6 Absence of a typical RBBB or LBBB pattern is suggestive of VT
7 Presence of AV dissociation, capture beats and fusion beats indicate VT
8 Very broad QRS complex (>150 ms) is indicative of VT
9 Concordance observed in the precordial or chest leads is called the 'either or' phenomenon in that all the leads either show positive complexes with predominant R waves

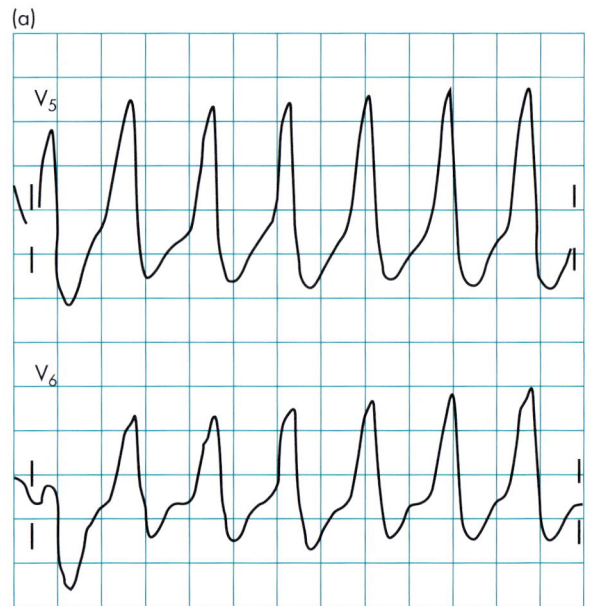
(a)

or negative complexes with QS waves (you do not see RS complexes).

10 When there is a positive complex in V_1 (and V_2) the first R wave is bigger than the second r wave in VT, as shown in Figure 2.7(b). This is also called the 'rabbit ear sign', a very specific sign in that the RSr complex in VT shows a 'taller left rabbit ear'. In RBBB with SVT, the 'right rabbit ear is taller' giving a rSR pattern.

11 In VT the QRS complex in V_4–V_6 is predominantly negative, and QR or QS complexes are seen in the leads V_2–V_6 (in both LBBB pattern and RBBB pattern VT).

12 In VT when there is a negative complex in V_1, there is a notch near the nadir of the S wave giving it a slurred appearance (Fig 2.7(c)).

MONOMORPHIC VT

Causes of monomorphic VT (Fig 2.7(a)) include:

- Coronary ischaemia or acute myocardial infarction
- Scar tissue in the myocardium (due to previous infarction)
- Heart failure
- Cardiomyopathy (dilated or hypertrophic)
- Drug toxicity, usually anti-arrhythmic agents (or digoxin in Wolff-Parkinson-White syndrome)
- Congenital syndromes, such as idiopathic VT of the young, right ventricular outflow tract (RVOT) VT, left ventricular outflow tract (LVOT) VT, right ventricular dysplasia, Brugada syndrome.

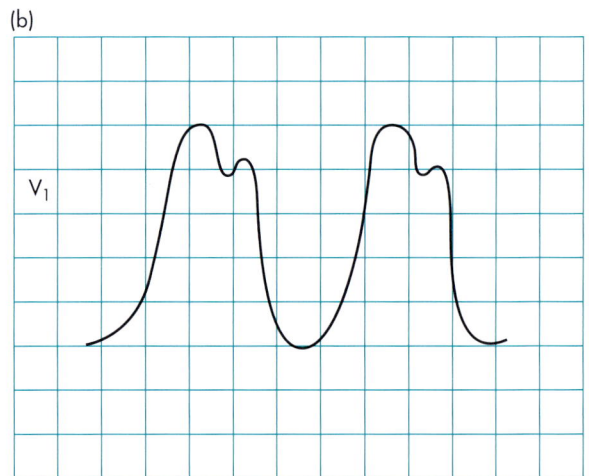
(b)

Presentation

Usually the patient presents with syncope, sudden cardiac death (cardiac arrest) or palpitations (conscious VT).

Acute management

The objective is to restore sinus rhythm and haemodynamic stability. If the patient is unconscious or in haemodynamic collapse, urgent DC electrical cardioversion should be

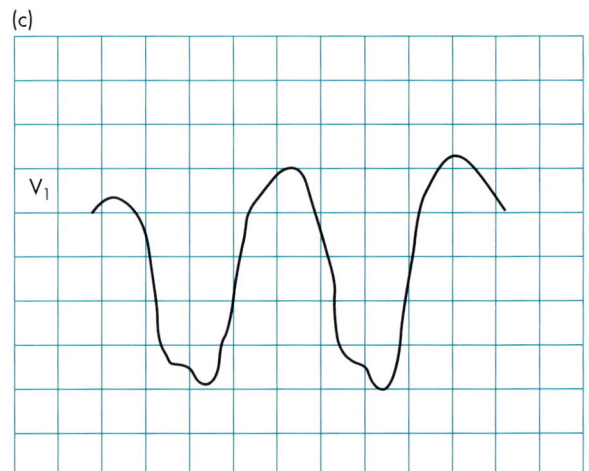
(c)

Figure 2.7 Ventricular tachycardia: (a) VT; (b) VT with 'taller left rabbit ear' in V_1 (RBBB); (c) VT with notch in the nadir of S wave (LBBB)

administered. Note that if there is a pulse you should cardiovert the patient with synchronisation (by pressing the 'synch' button on the defibrillator device). The starting energy for VT with pulse is 200 J, but for biphasic devices this can be 120 J.

If there is no pulse then deliver a defibrillator shock without synchronisation. The same strategy should be adopted for VF: the first shock in VF or pulseless VT should be 360 J for monophasic devices and 150 J for biphasic devices. Shock energy should be increased up to 360 J if the lower energy shocks fail to restore sinus rhythm.

If there is evidence of coronary ischaemia as a precipitant, a lignocaine infusion should be commenced along with urgent measures to reopen the closed coronary artery by thrombolysis or by primary percutaneous intervention (primary angioplasty).

Magnesium or potassium deficiency can lead to VT, so check the patient's magnesium and potassium levels and give replacement of these electrolytes. Magnesium infusion may be beneficial even if the serum magnesium levels are normal.

Other drugs to be used in this situation include amiodarone and procainamide.

Long-term management

To prevent recurrent events it is important to address the causative factors adequately. These measures include coronary revascularisation (angioplasty or bypass surgery as required), treating heart failure, replacing deficient electrolytes or removing the offending drug if it is due to drug toxicity.

Drugs that can be used to prevent VT include beta-blockers, amiodarone and sotalol.

Catheter radiofrequency ablation is possible for some types of VT, such as RVOT or LVOT origin VT, and scar associated VT. The last is a complex procedure requiring operator expertise and experience, together with specialised mapping equipment and catheters.

Those who are at high risk of recurrent cardiac arrest should be managed with an implanted cardiac defibrillator (ICD).

POLYMORPHIC VT (TORSADES DE POINTES)

The QRS complexes in this type of VT show change in morphology with the axis shifting or twisting between two opposing points (Fig 2.8). Hence the complexes show upward deflection first

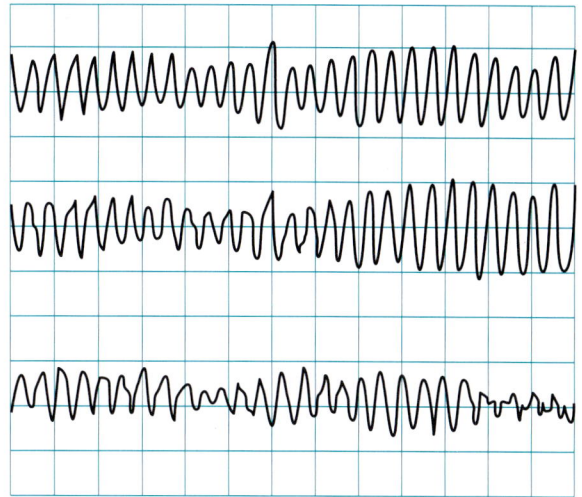

Figure 2.8 Torsades de pointes

then gradually change to downward deflection, and this shifting of the axis keeps happening in a sequential manner. The ventricle is stimulated by impulses originating from two different foci within the ventricle itself.

Torsades de pointes is usually triggered by a premature ventricular complex (PVC). Torsades can rapidly degenerate into ventricular fibrillation, so urgent intervention is required. Rapid torsades can lead to haemodynamic compromise and syncope.

Torsades can be caused by several different factors. Many drugs that can prolong the QT interval can cause torsades. Some such agents include macrolide antibiotics, antihistamines, tricyclic antidepressants, lithium and anti-arrhythmics such as quinidine, procainamide and sotalol. Other causes include congenital long QT syndrome, hypoxaemia, hypothermia, bradycardia, electrolyte abnormalities and myocardial ischaemia. The commonly associated electrolyte abnormalities are hypomagnesaemia, hypokalaemia and hypocalcaemia.

Management of torsades

If a causative factor can be identified it should be removed or remedied and, if the patient is unstable, urgent DC unsynchronised electric cardioversion or defibrillation should be carried out. Other treatment modalities in the stable patient include magnesium sulfate infusion and anti-arrhythmic agents, such as mexiletine. Magnesium infusion (at 3–10 milligrams per min) is useful even when the serum magnesium level is normal.

The tachycardia can be terminated by a faster rhythm that overrides it. Such a rhythm can be chemically induced with an isoprenaline infusion. It can also be induced with a temporary pacemaker programmed to pace at a higher rate, called 'overdrive pacing'.

ACCELERATED IDIOVENTRICULAR RHYTHM

By definition this is a ventricular escape rhythm that is faster than 40 bpm (the intrinsic rate of ventricular depolarisation). This rhythm has a rate slower than ventricular tachycardia. Thus accelerated idioventricular rhythm usually has a rate of 40–120 bpm with more than three beats occurring sequentially. The causative factors include myocardial ischaemia, reopening of a blocked coronary artery after thrombolysis or angioplasty (reperfusion arrhythmia), digoxin toxicity and heart failure. The 12-lead ECG tracing may show AV dissociation, capture beats and fusion beats indicating the ventricular origin of the rhythm. This rhythm is usually well tolerated by the patient and often self terminates.

Ventricular flutter

This is ventricular tachycardia with a rate of over 200 bpm. The ECG tracing indicates a sinusoidal rhythm, a very unstable rhythm that degenerates rapidly into ventricular fibrillation and cardiac arrest (Fig 2.9).

Ventricular fibrillation

A disorganised and chaotic rhythm arising from multiple foci within the ventricle. The disorganised nature of this rhythm makes it impossible to facilitate effective ventricular contraction to maintain a cardiac output. VF can rapidly cause cardiac arrest and death. Treatment is to initiate cardiopulmonary resuscitation and urgent electrical defibrillation.

BRADYARRHYTHMIAS AND BRADYCARDIA

When the heart rate is less than 50 bpm it is called bradycardia. It may be due to multiple causes, both pathological and physiological. Sinus bradycardia is signified by normal P waves with QRS complexes of normal duration. Haemodynamically tolerated bradycardia (with no hypotension or syncopal symptoms) is due to vagal overdrive and usually seen in well-trained athletes. Bradycardia due to vagal overdrive is also

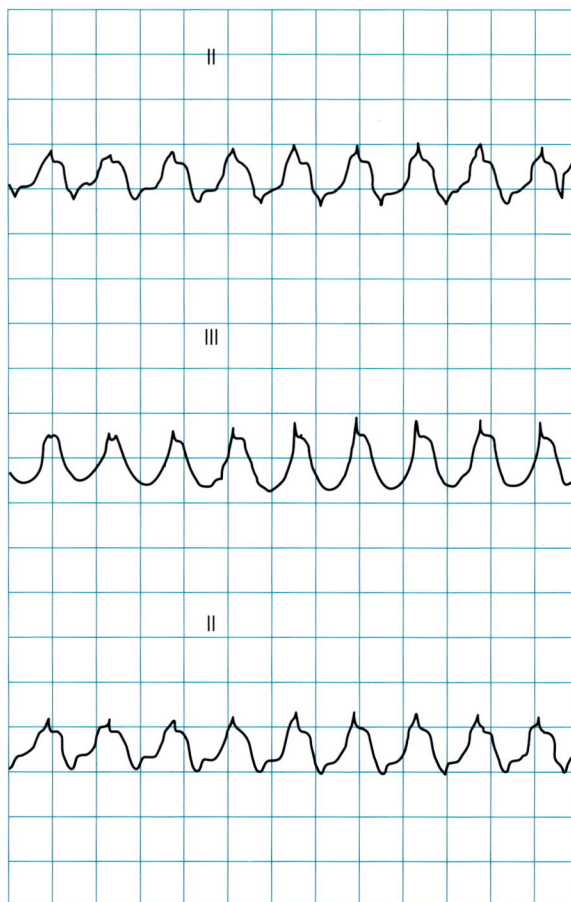

Figure 2.9 Ventricular flutter

seen during sleep. Drugs that act on the SA node, such as ivabradine, and those that act on the AV node, such as beta-blockers, calcium channel blockers and digoxin, can also cause bradycardia. Other causes of bradyarrhythmias include hyperkalaemia, hypothermia, coronary ischaemia and shock.

The conduction defect or the block that gives rise to the bradyarrhythmia could be at any level in the conduction system: SA node, AV node, bundle of His, left bundle branch or right bundle branch. Therefore the classification of bradyarrhythmias is based on the location of the conduction block.

Block at the level of the SA node

Sinus arrest

Sinus arrest is the failure of the SA node to fire for a period of 3 seconds or more. The causative factors are as described above for bradycardia.

ECG can show prolonged pauses with absent P waves. In the absence of an SA nodal impulse, the QRS complexes are generated at the AV node or below. Usually a prolonged pause appears on the ECG followed by a normal looking P wave, and a QRS complex if the SA node recovers. At times the rhythm may be irregular with an appearance that is similar to complete heart block.

Sinoatrial exit block (SA block)

This arrhythmia is due to the intermittent failure of the SA node impulse to conduct to the right atrium. The PP interval will gradually shorten in consecutive beats until a pause occurs. The pause is shorter than two PP intervals in length. After the pause the conduction resumes again.

Block at the level of the AV node

First degree heart block (1st degree AV block)

In this situation the PR interval is longer than 200 ms (Fig 2.10(a)). Every P wave is conducted to the ventricle as the block is located in the AV node. This situation needs no specific therapy provided the patient is maintaining a satisfactory heart rate.

Second degree heart block (2nd degree AV block)

Not all impulses from the sinoatrial node are conducted to the ventricles. There are two types as follows:

1 Type 1, 2nd degree HB, also called the Wenckebach phenomenon

The PR interval is prolonged gradually until a beat or a P wave is skipped or not conducted to the ventricle (Fig 2.10(b)). The block is always located in the AV node. This situation does not require any specific therapy.

2 Type 2, 2nd degree HB

The PR interval remains normal and constant until one P waves fails to conduct to the ventricle. This causes a pause and another P wave to appear before the next QRS complex (Fig 2.10(c)). The block is located in the bundle branches, hence the QRS complex may appear wider.

If only one in two sinus impulses (P waves) is conducted to the ventricle, it is called a two to one block. When only one in three impulses (P waves) is conducted, it is a three to one block. Usually this condition can progress to complete heart block, so it requires therapy with the implantation of a pacemaker if no other reversible cause (such as electrolyte abnormality or negatively chronotropic drug therapy) is identified and corrected.

Third degree heart block (complete heart block)

None of the sinus impulses are conducted to the ventricle (Fig 2.10(d)). Ventricular excitation is due to impulses generated at the level of the AV node (nodal rhythm) or at the level of the ventricles (idioventricular rhythm). The QRS complex appears wider when it is idioventricular in origin. Both these rhythms are slower than sinus rhythm and have the potential to cause severe life-threatening bradycardia. The blockage could be at the AV node (most commonly) or the bundle of His. This condition requires the implantation of a pacemaker. Until a permanent pacemaker can be implanted, the patient could be stabilised on an isoprenaline infusion or with the help of a transvenous temporary pacemaker.

ABNORMALITIES OF THE CARDIAC RHYTHM

Normal cardiac rhythm is regular. Irregularity of the rhythm is usually due to a pathology. Pathological rhythm irregularities can be 'regularly irregular' or 'irregularly irregular'. The regularly irregular rhythms have a recurrent set pattern while irregularly irregular rhythm is usually chaotic.

Regularly irregular rhythms

- Sinus arrhythmia — small changes in heart rate occur with breathing in and out. This is a normal observation, usually seen in healthy children and young adults
- Second degree heart block.

Irregularly irregular rhythms

- AF
- Multifocal ectopic beats — atrial or ventricular
- Complete heart block (but not always).

THE P WAVE

The P wave represents the sum of sequential activation of the right atrium and then the left atrium. Due to this, the P wave at times can

(a) First degree heart block

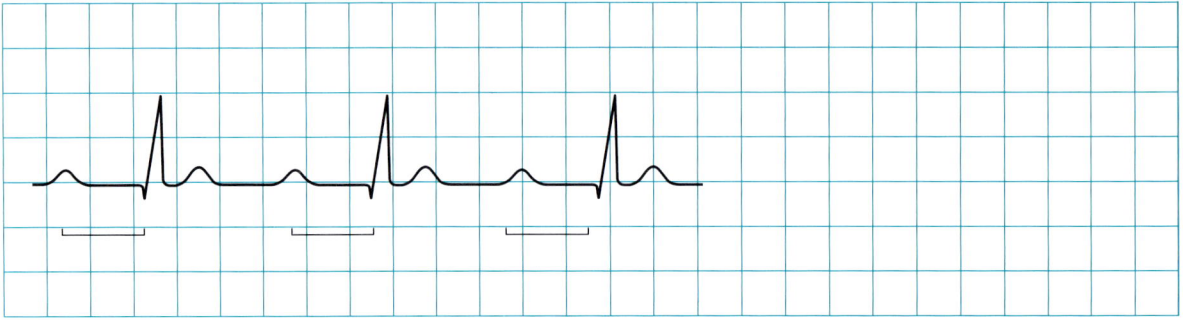

(b) Second degree heart block type 1

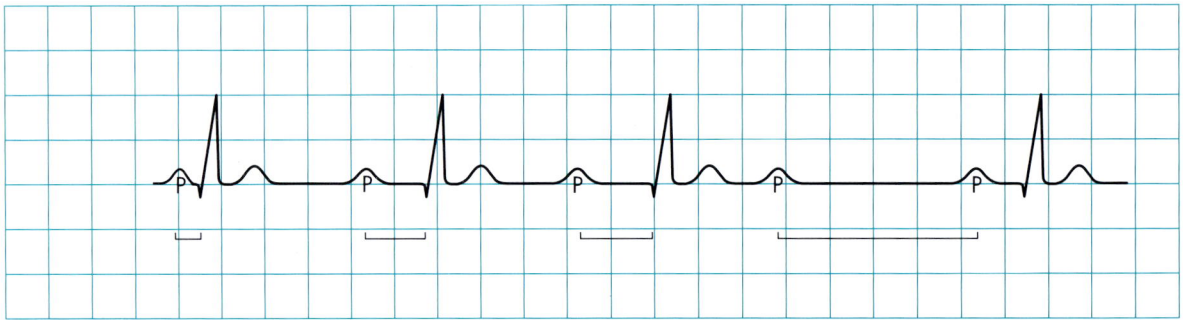

(c) Second degree heart block type 2 3:1

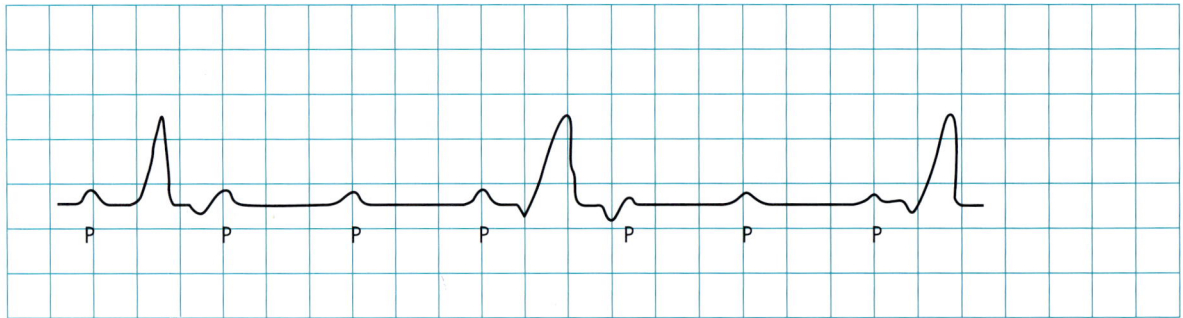

(d) Third degree heart block

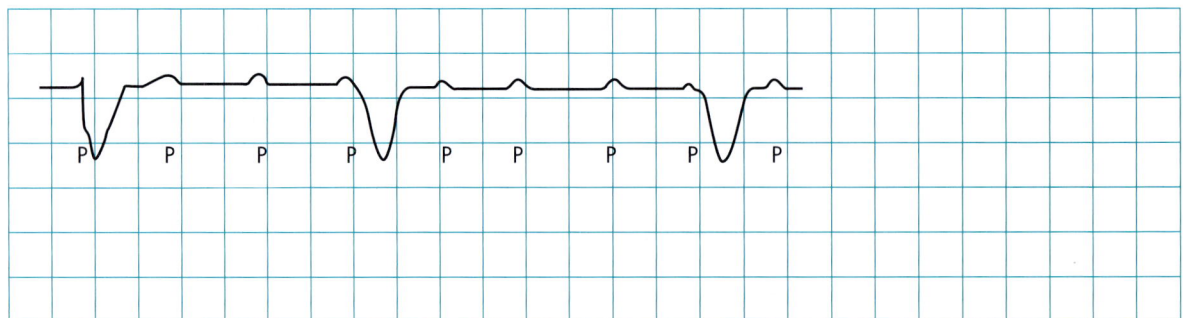

Figure 2.10 Different types of heart block: (a) first degree heart block, note the long PR interval; (b) second degree heart block, type I, note the gradual prolongation of PR interval until one P wave is skipped; (c) second degree heart block, type 2; (d) third degree heart block

appear notched or biphasic (with both upward and downward deflections). Its axis on the frontal plane is between 0° and 75°. The wave is usually less than 120 ms in duration and less than 2.5 mm in amplitude.

Abnormalities of the P wave

Absent P wave

The P wave could be absent in AF, idioventricular rhythm, VT and junctional rhythm.

Abnormal P wave morphology

Changes in the amplitude or morphology of the P wave can be associated with:

1 Right atrial enlargement (RAE)

The P wave appears tall; this is also called P-pulmonale. The height of the P wave is more than 2.5 mm in lead II, and more than 1.5 mm in V_1.

2 Left atrial enlargement (LAE)

The P wave is long and notched. In lead II the P wave duration can be observed to be more than 120 ms. Note the notching of the P wave in the limb leads.

3 Biatrial enlargement (BAE)

The P wave is both tall and elongated with a notch; the previously described features of RAE and LAE are present in the same ECG. The P wave in lead II is more than 2.5 mm tall with duration longer than 120 ms.

THE PR INTERVAL

- Prolonged PR interval — The prolongation of the PR interval is seen in first degree heart block
- Shortened PR interval — An abnormally short (less than 200 ms) PR interval is seen in pre-excitation syndromes such as Wolff-Parkinson-White (WPW) syndrome and Lown-Ganong-Levine (LGL) syndrome.

LGL syndrome

LGL syndrome is characterised by a very short PR interval, less than 120 ms, but in contrast to WPW syndrome there is no delta wave in the QRS complex. The accessory pathway connects atrial tissue to the bundle of His. Just like WPW syndrome, this too can lead to AVNRT. When the atria are beating fast, the rapidly conducted impulses along the accessory pathway can lead to dangerous and fatal malignant tachyarrhythmia.

This syndrome is considered to have a rather benign course compared to that of WPW syndrome. SVT associated with this pathology can be treated with beta-blockers or calcium channel blockers. When drug therapy fails, AV node ablation and the implantation of a pacemaker may be indicated.

THE PR SEGMENT

The PR segment is usually isoelectric, so it lies on the baseline. PR depression or elevation can indicate atrial pathology.

Atrial ischaemia can cause the PR segment to shift. Observation of PR segment elevation or depression can be seen in myocardial infarctions. This is due to atrial ischaemia. Observation of PR segment depression in myocardial infarction indicates a worse prognosis.

Acute pericarditis can be associated with PR segment depression.

THE QRS COMPLEX

The various elements of the QRS complex represent the sequential depolarisation of the right ventricle and then the left ventricle. However the representation of the left ventricular depolarisation predominates the QRS morphology. Usually its duration is less than 120 ms. However the amplitude (represented by the height) and the duration (represented by the width) can vary due to various reasons. The main factors affecting the amplitude are the thickness of the ventricular wall (degree of hypertrophy) and the proximity of the heart to the chest wall.

The QRS complex is mostly positive and upright in leads I and II. The normal QRS axis is between +90° and −30°.

Q wave

A normal Q wave (initial negative deflection) is less than 40 ms wide and less than 25 per cent of the length of the following R wave (usually less than 0.1 mm deep). A Q wave is prominent in the lead aVR in a normal ECG, because the depolarisation wave travels from right to left.

- A small Q (called 'q') wave is clearly seen in leads I and aVL when the cardiac axis is deviated to the left, that is left of +60°.
- A small q wave is seen in leads II and III when the axis is deviated to the right, that is right of +60°.
- Small q waves are seen in V_5 and V_6 due to septal depolarisation.

- Pathological Q waves are seen after a transmural myocardial infarction; they are usually larger than 25 per cent of the R wave that follows, hence they are called significant.

R wave

Normally the R wave is small in V_1 and V_2 (called 'r'). It increases in its amplitude gradually from V_3 to V_4 and V_5. Absence of this gradual increment in the amplitude of the R wave is called poor R wave progression. The R wave in V_6 is slightly smaller than that in V_5.

S wave

The S wave is small in V_1 and becomes longer in V_2, then from V_2 to V_5 its amplitude gradually decreases.

Abnormalities in the height or depth of the QRS complex vertically or in its width horizontally can indicate a possible underlying pathology.

Widened QRS complex

A QRS complex wider than 120 ms (three small squares) is seen in:

1. Bundle branch blocks — left bundle branch block (LBBB) or right bundle branch block (RBBB)
2. Ventricular pacemaker rhythm
3. Pre-excitation in WPW syndrome (delta wave)
4. Ventricular rhythm
5. Hyperkalaemia.

Complete LBBB

The features of left bundle branch block (see Fig 2.11) are:

- Wide QRS complex with a duration of more than 120 ms
- Prominent and wide R waves in leads V_5, V_6, aVL and I
- Prominent S wave or QS complex in lead V_1
- Poor R wave progression in leads V_1 to V_3
- ST segment depression in the above leads with T wave inversion (discordant ST segment shift).

Note: LBBB is almost always pathological. A new LBBB with chest pain can indicate acute myocardial infarction with the occlusion of the left coronary artery. Other causes include fibrotic degeneration (also called Lev's disease), chronic hypertension and cardiomyopathy.

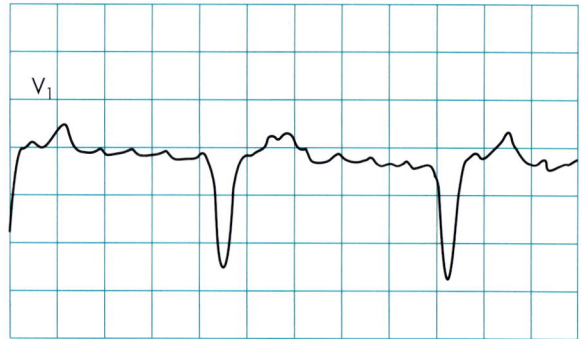

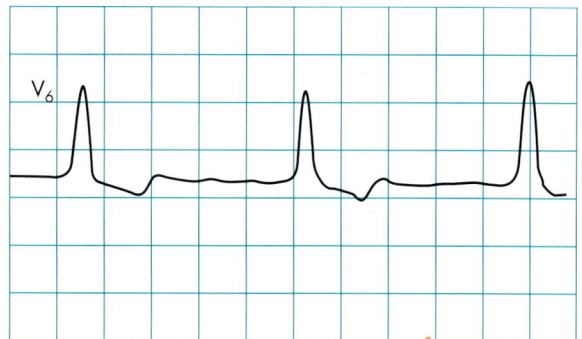

Figure 2.11 Left bundle branch block

Incomplete LBBB

The left bundle has two branches or fascicles, anterior and posterior. When only one fascicle is blocked, it is called incomplete LBBB. The QRS duration is slightly prolonged. It is usually seen in LVH.

Left anterior fascicular block (LAFB)

This is more common than posterior fascicular block. Features are:

- Axis is deviated to the left between −90° and −45°
- Small q waves in leads I and/or aVL
- Small r waves in inferior leads (II, III and aVF) together with prominent S waves (rS complexes in inferior leads)
- Deep S waves in leads V_5 and V_6
- There may be poor R wave progression in leads V_1 to V_3.

Left posterior fascicular block (LPFB)

- Axis is deviated to the right to more than +100°
- Prominent S wave in lead I and the anterior chest leads (leads V_3 and V_4)

- Small r waves in the lateral leads, rS in leads 1 and aVL
- Prominent R waves together with small q waves in leads II, III and aVF — the qR pattern. Note that the R wave in lead III may be taller than that in lead II.

BIFASCICULAR BLOCKS

When two conduction pathways in the heart are blocked, it is called bifascicular block. They may be:

1 LAFB together with RBBB

The more common form, where the ECG features of RBBB together with left axis deviation are seen.

2 LPFB together with RBBB

When features of RBBB and right axis deviation are observed, the possibility of RBBB and LPFB should be considered.

Right bundle branch block

Features of RBBB (Fig 2.12) are:

- The duration of the QRS complex is longer than 120 ms

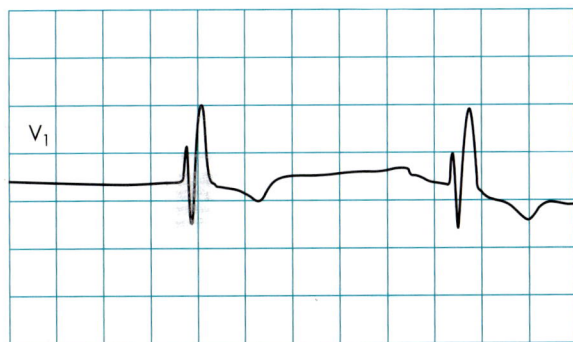

- Axis remains within normal limits (between $-30°$ and $+90°$)
- The rSR pattern is in lead V_1 with a prominent second R wave after the S wave
- Terminal S waves in leads I, aVL and V_6
- A qRS complex in lead V_6
- A terminal R wave also in lead aVR
- T wave inversion and ST segment depression can be seen in V_1 and aVR
- ST segment elevation can sometimes be seen in leads V_5 and/or V_6.

If the QRS duration is prolonged with no specific features of LBBB or RBBB present, it is called a non-specific intraventricular conduction defect (IVCD). This is observed in acute myocardial infarction, AMI, in the presence of anti-arrhythmic drugs, such as flecainide or quinidine, and in WPW syndrome.

WOLFF-PARKINSON-WHITE SYNDROME

This syndrome develops due to the presence of an accessory pathway that connects atria to the ventricles. This pathway is called the bundle of Kent. The QRS complex is widened in WPW syndrome due to the stimulation or excitation of the ventricle by two different pathways simultaneously: the AV nodal pathway and the bundle of Kent. This causes the characteristic slurring of the QRS complex, and this additional deflection of the QRS complex is called the delta wave (Fig 2.13). The delta wave represents the early activation of the ventricle by the accessory pathway. The other feature of WPW pre-excitation is the short PR interval, usually less than 120 ms.

- The QRS complex duration is prolonged due to the delta wave

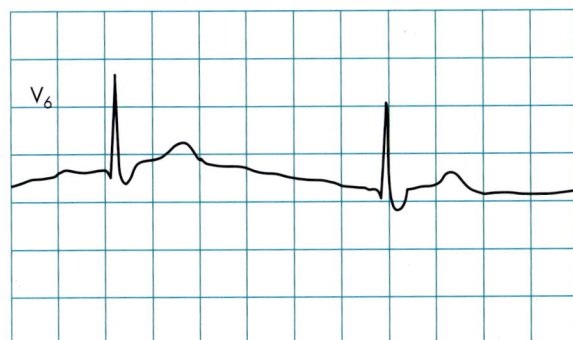

Figure 2.12 Right bundle branch block

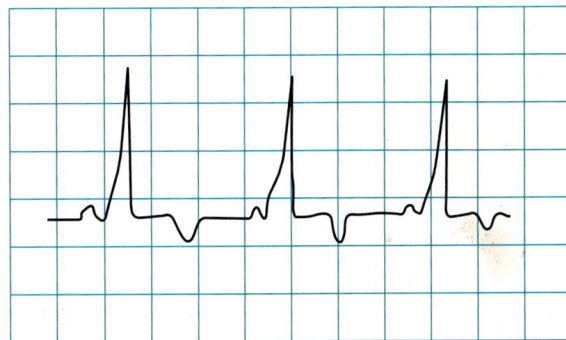

Figure 2.13 Wolff-Parkinson-White syndrome: note the short PR interval and the delta wave

- There may be secondary ST segment and T wave changes associated with abnormalities in the repolarisation process.

Estimation of the location of the accessory pathway in WPW syndrome

The location of the accessory pathway can be predicted by observing the axis of the ECG and the morphology of the QRS complex in leads V_1 and V_2. This determination is useful for locating the anatomical position of the accessory pathway for therapeutic radiofrequency ablation.

- If the QRS complexes in V_1 and V_2 have predominantly positive deflections (dominant R waves with delta waves) together with left axis deviation, the pathway is in the posterior aspect of the interventricular septum in the left side. This is called type A WPW pre-excitation or 'positive delta WPW syndrome' due to the positive delta wave in V_1.

- If the QRS complex is negatively deflected in V_1 and V_2 (dominant QS waves with delta waves) with a left axis deviation, the pathway is in the right ventricle in the lateral aspect. This is called type B or 'negative delta WPW syndrome' due to the negative delta wave in V_1.

- If the QRS complex is deflected upwards (positively) in both V_1 and V_2 with an inferior axis ($+90°$), the accessory pathway is in the left ventricular wall laterally: this is called type C.

- If the QRS complex is negatively deflected in both V_1 and V_2 with a leftward axis, the accessory pathway is in the right posteroseptal region.

- If the QRS complex is negatively deflected in both V_1 and V_2 with a normal axis, the accessory pathway is in the anteroseptal region.

- In general, if there is positive deflection in leads V_1 and V_2, the pathway is in the left side. If it is negatively deflected it is in the right side (if the axis is leftward).

Clinical points on WPW syndrome

Patients with WPW can present with presyncope, syncope, palpitations and dyspnoea. People with WPW can develop AVRT and AF. The dreaded consequence of WPW is sudden death due to a rapid atrial rhythm conducting to the ventricle via the accessory pathway with no rate control (usually brought about by the AV node) leading to VT and VF. This can be caused by drugs that block the AV node, such as digoxin, calcium channel blockers and beta-blockers. These drugs should be avoided in WPW syndrome. AF in WPW should be treated with amiodarone, procainamide or DC cardioversion. Those patients at high risk of sudden death or recurrent symptoms need electrophysiological investigation and radiofrequency ablation of the bundle of Kent.

VENTRICULAR ECTOPIC BEATS

Ventricular ectopic beats (VEBs) are characterised by occasional broad QRS complexes that occur in the presence of a supraventricular rhythm. These complexes differ in morphology to the QRS complexes of the underlying rhythm. They are not preceded by a P wave indicating their ventricular origin. The types of VEBs are:

1 Salvos — bursts of repetitive ventricular ectopy
2 Couplet — two successive VEBs
3 Triplet — three successive VEBs (Fig 2.14)
4 Quadruplets — four successive VEBs.

Idioventricular rhythm (ventricular escape rhythm)

This is a rhythm originating in a secondary ventricular pacemaker that becomes the dominant rhythm when there is no faster supraventricular

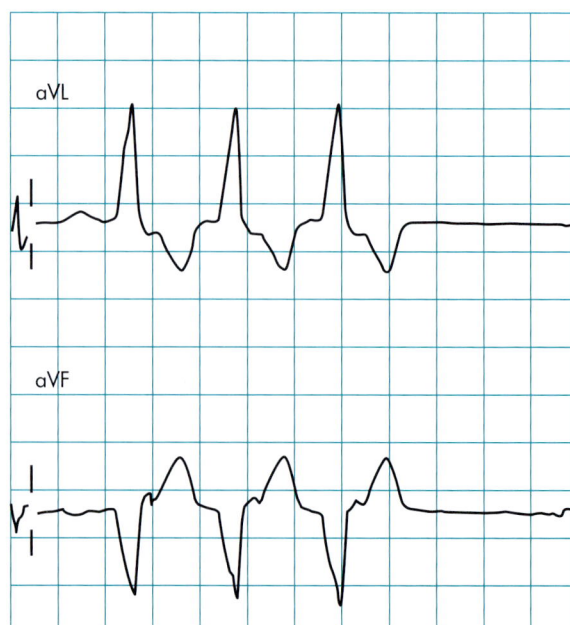

Figure 2.14 A triplet

rhythm present. The QRS complexes are uniform in morphology and very broad (>140 ms). They are not preceded by a P wave. The rate is 30–45 bpm. If the rate is faster than 60 bpm (up to 120 bpm), it is called accelerated idioventricular rhythm. This rhythm is so defined if more than three consecutive ventricular beats occur at this rate.

ABERRANCY

Aberrancy is a conduction defect located in the ventricular level. This phenomenon is characterised by a broad QRS complex.

Abnormalities in the height of the QRS complex

Abnormalities in the height of the QRS complex can signify underlying pathology. Some of these anatomical cardiac abnormalities manifested on ECG are discussed below.

Left ventricular hypertrophy (LVH)

This is caused by chronic hypertension or chronic aortic stenosis. Rarely does LVH develop due to genetic mutations that are inherited or de novo. Physical examination will reveal an apical heave. Tall R waves in the lateral (LV) leads and deep S waves in the right-sided (RV) leads are characteristic of LVH (Fig 2.15). ECG changes are of very low sensitivity (<50%) but of high specificity (>90%) for the diagnosis of LVH.

ECG FEATURES OF LVH

There are two sets of criteria for the diagnosis of LVH on ECG. The first is the voltage criteria based on the amplitude of the R waves and S waves in specific leads as discussed below. The second is the strain criteria based on the changes in ST segment and T waves in the respective leads.

1 Voltage criteria of LVH

- Left axis deviation
- Tall R waves in V_5 and V_6 (height of more than 2.5 cm)
- Deep S waves in V_1 and V_2 (depth of usually more than 3 cm)
- The combined length of the S wave in V_1 and the R wave in V_5 or V_6 is more than 3.5 cm
- Tall R waves in lead aVL (of more than 1.1 cm)
- Deep S waves in lead III (of more than 1.5 cm).

In LVH all or some of the above features may be present be on the ECG. The more criteria that are present the more likely the diagnosis.

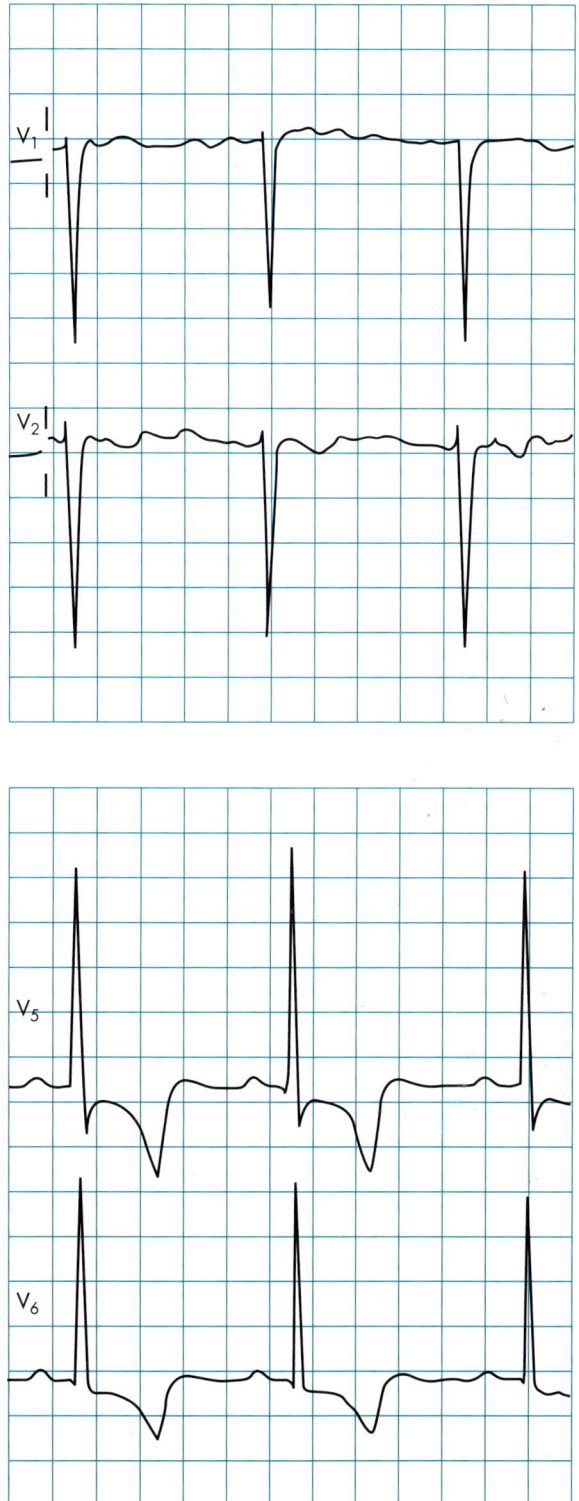

Figure 2.15 Left ventricular hypertrophy

2 Strain criteria of LVH

- T wave inversion and ST segment depression in leads V_5 and V_6 (in the absence of digitalis effect).

Right ventricular hypertrophy (RVH)

This is seen in pathologies such as pulmonary valve stenosis, pulmonary hypertension and/or chronic lung disease. When the RVH is due to lung pathology, it is called cor pulmonale. Physical examination will reveal a parasternal heave suggesting the RVH.

ECG FEATURES OF RVH

- Right axis deviation (axis directed at >100°)
- Tall R waves in lead V_1 (>6–7 mm) with a smaller s wave of less than 2 mm, that is, the R wave is more than twice the height of the s wave in V_1
- rSR pattern in the QRS complex in lead V_1 with the second R wave taller than 1 cm
- Tall R wave in lead aVR of >5 mm or the R wave is longer than the Q wave in aVR
- Dominant (deep) S waves in V_6 (and V_5 often), usually >7 mm, so the S wave is larger than the R wave in V_6
- T wave inversion in lead V_1
- T wave inversion in leads V_2 and V_3
- ST/T wave changes directed in the opposite direction to that of QRS complex.

Biventricular hypertrophy

The changes of biventricular hypertrophy are a combination of features seen in LVH and RVH. Biventricular hypertrophy can also be represented on an ECG by features of LVH together with right axis deviation.

Other changes to note include:

- Deep S waves in V_5 and/or V_6 of more than 5 mm
- R/S ratio of leads V_5 and/or V_6 of less than 1

QRS morphology

Changes in QRS morphology can be summarised as:

- Widening of the QRS complex — see RBBB and LBBB
- Delta wave — see WPW syndrome
- rSR pattern — seen in RBBB.

THE ST SEGMENT

The ST segment is the horizontal line between the end of the S wave, at a point called the J (junctional) point, and the beginning of the T wave. The ST segment normally is isoelectric and remains at the baseline. It can be elevated without any underlying pathology in leads V_1 to V_3, especially when the S wave is large: this is called high take-off.

The ST segment normally lies within the baseline, and elevation or depression may indicate an underlying pathology if there are complementary clinical features. Dynamic changes or shifts in the ST segment that vary over time are more significant than fixed changes. These could suggest an underlying unstable clinical condition, such as acute coronary ischaemia. Those changes in the ST segment that do not corroborate a clinical finding are called non-specific changes.

ST segment shift

An ST segment shift from baseline can be due to the following pathologies:

1. Coronary ischaemia
2. Myocarditis or pericarditis
3. Left ventricular aneurysm
4. Drug effects from digoxin, tricyclic antidepressants or quinidine
5. Conduction abnormalities within the ventricles
6. Acute subarachnoid haemorrhage
7. Takotsubo cardiomyopathy
8. Brugada syndrome
9. Electrolyte abnormality.

ST segment changes can be a result of other more specific ECG diagnoses, called secondary ST segment changes. Some situations of secondary changes in the ST segment are:

- Intraventricular conduction defects, such as bundle branch block or fascicular block
- Ventricular paced rhythm
- In pre-excitation, such as in WPW syndrome
- Hypertrophy of the ventricles.

ST segment elevation

ST segment elevation can indicate several underlying cardiac pathologies. It may be a normal phenomenon when there are no associated clinical features to suggest a pathology. The various causes of ST segment elevation are:

1 Early repolarisation of the ventricles can cause ST segment elevation, and is called high take-off. The elevated ST segment has a concave upward morphology and is followed by a large T wave. Usually the patient remains asymptomatic. Typically the ST segment elevation is less than 2 mm in the anteroseptal leads and less than 1 mm in the inferior leads.

2 Acute pericarditis where ST segment elevation has a concavity facing upward (Fig 2.16(a)). It is usually seen in all leads, perhaps except for in aVR. There is also PR segment depression suggesting inflammation in the atrial regions. But it can rarely be localised to a specific region of the heart, with ST segment shift seen only in the leads representing this zone. Acute pericarditis presents with pleuritic chest pain that is sharp in character and exacerbates with leaning forward. On examination there is a 'pericardial friction rub' audible, especially when leaning forward.

3 Acute transmural myocardial infarction where the morphology of the elevated ST segment is convex upward (Fig 2.16(b)). This feature is also called the 'tombstone' ST elevation due to the nature of the underlying pathology.

4 Left ventricular aneurysm can cause ST segment elevation. If the ST segment elevation persists after a myocardial infarction, the formation of an aneurysm in the infarcted section of the myocardium should be suspected. This can be confirmed by echocardiography. Very often there is mural thrombus formation within the LV cavity at the aneurysm, so these patients require therapeutic anticoagulation with warfarin.

5 ST segment elevation, which is transient or dynamic, can be seen with Prinzmetal's angina, also called variant angina. It is due to coronary artery spasm.

6 ST segment elevation seen during exercise stress testing can be suggestive of a tight stenosis of the left main coronary artery or the proximal left anterior descending (LAD) artery.

7 ST segment elevation can be a secondary change associated with LVH or LBBB.

8 ST segment elevation in the septal leads mimicking left anterior descending artery territory infarction is seen in Takotsubo cardiomyopathy. This is an acute event seen mostly in middle-aged females subjected to significant psychological or emotional trauma. The pathology is related to a sudden adrenergic surge in the circulation that is believed to lead to coronary ischaemia, often in a normal appearing non-occluded coronary tree.

Anterolateral myocardial infarction

- There is a convex upward ST segment elevation in leads V_4 to V_6 of more than 2 mm, making it significant. Associated ST segment elevation is also seen in leads I and aVL that represent the left side of the heart.

- In this case the blocked vessel is likely to be the LAD artery that supplies the septal and anterior regions of the left ventricle, with the associated flow limitation in the diagonal branches supplying blood to the lateral wall. The occlusion is likely to be located at a point proximal to the origin of the diagonal branch.

- When the infarction zone is limited to the anterior wall of the LV and the interventricular septum, the ST segment elevation is seen in

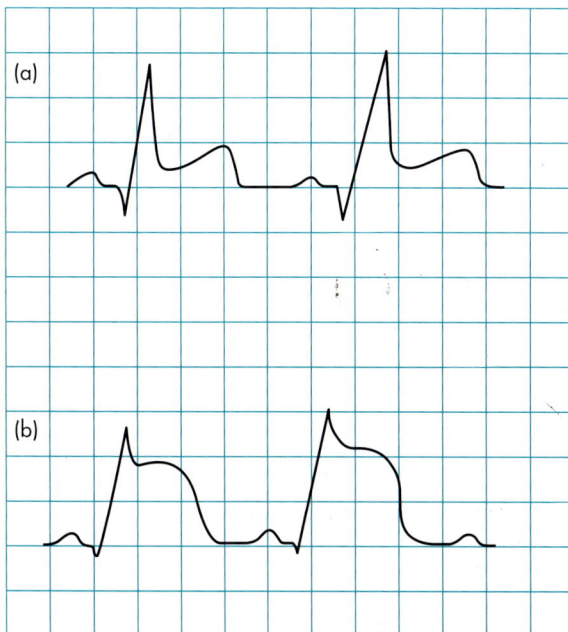

Figure 2.16 ST segment elevation: (a) concave up as in pericarditis; (b) convex up as seen in acute myocardial infarction

leads V_2, V_3 and perhaps V_4 only. The blocked artery once again is the LAD but distal to the origin of the major diagonal branch that supplies the lateral wall.

- When only the lateral wall is infarcting, the ST segment elevation of more than 2 mm is seen in leads V_5 and V_6 together with leads I and aVL; all these leads represent the lateral wall of the left ventricle. The culprit artery here could be the left circumflex artery or a dominant diagonal branch of the LAD artery.

Inferior wall myocardial infarction

In inferior wall myocardial infarction, ST segment elevation of more than 1 mm is seen in leads II, III and aVF. There may be corresponding reciprocal ST segment depression seen in the leads V_1, V_2 and V_3. The culprit vessel is a dominant right coronary artery in 90 per cent of the population, however in the other 10 per cent it is caused by the occlusion of a dominant left circumflex branch.

Right ventricular (RV) infarction

- Usually right ventricular STEMI (ST elevation myocardial infarction) is associated with inferior wall STEMI because both regions are supplied by the right coronary artery in the majority of the population. If the occlusion is proximal to the origin of the right ventricular branch, there will be RV involvement. RV infarction is suggested by ST segment elevation in the leads V_1, V_2 and/or V_3 usually in the setting of ST segment elevation in the inferior leads. Sometimes there is ST segment depression in leads V_1, V_2 and V_3.
- A right-sided ECG should be performed in this case. There will be ST segment elevation in V_4R, V_5R and V_6R. ST segment elevation of more than 1 mm in V_4R is highly sensitive and absolutely specific for RV infarction. Hence, if you see significant ST segment elevation in these leads in the setting of inferior infarct, it is important to obtain the V_4R tracing.

Posterior wall myocardial infarction

Posterior wall myocardial infarction is rare and is usually associated with infarction of other regions of the left ventricle. It is more commonly associated with inferior MI. Clues to suspect posterior wall MI include:

- ST segment depression in the leads V_1, V_2 and V_3 with deep T wave inversion, with the changes more prominent in lead V_2.
- An important feature is the R/S ratio that is greater than 1 (R wave longer than the S wave) in the leads V_1, V_2 and V_3.
- There could be late normalisation of the ST segment with tall, upright T waves in the leads V_1, V_2 and V_3.

A posterior ECG should be performed to confirm the diagnosis. The features of posterior MI in the posterior ECG include ST segment elevation in the leads V_7, V_8 and V_9.

ECG criteria for acute reperfusion therapy

ECG criteria for acute reperfusion therapy using thrombolysis or primary angioplasty:

- Anterolateral STEMI: ST segment elevation in the anterolateral leads (V_3 to V_6) of at least 2 mm in two adjacent leads.
- Inferior STEMI: More than 1 mm of ST segment elevation in at least two of the three inferior leads or II, III and aVF.
- New LBBB.

Summary notes on STEMI-associated ECG changes

- Septal infarct will show ST segment elevation in leads V_1, V_2 and V_3. Reciprocal ST segment depression will be seen in leads V_7, V_8 and V_9 (posterior).
- Anterior infarct will show ST segment elevation in the leads V_3 and V_4. Reciprocal ST segment depression will be seen in leads V_8 and V_9 (posterior).
- Lateral wall infarct will show ST segment elevation in leads V_5 and V_6.
- High lateral wall infarct will show ST segment elevation in the leads I and aVL. The reciprocal ST segment depression is seen in the leads II, III and aVF.
- Inferior wall infarct will show ST segment elevation in the leads II, III and aVF. Reciprocal ST segment depression is seen in the leads I and aVL.
- Right ventricular infarct is characterised by ST segment elevation in leads V_1, V_2 and V_3 with leads II and III. The degree of ST elevation in

lead III is bigger than that of lead II. In the right-sided ECG there is ST elevation in leads V_4R, V_5R and V_6R. Reciprocal ST segment depression is seen in lead V_2.

- Posterior wall infarct shows ST segment elevation in leads V_7, V_8 and V_9 (posterior leads). Reciprocal ST segment depression is seen in leads V_1, V_2 and V_3. The coronary artery involved is the posterior descending branch.

- ST segment elevation in the isolated lead of aVR is indicative of complete occlusion of the left main coronary artery.

CLINICAL NOTES ON STEMI

Usually the patient presents with chest tightness, diaphoresis and nausea. Delayed presentations can be with acute pulmonary oedema and cardiogenic shock. Some may present with cardiac arrest. The patient should be managed with urgent therapy to re-open the blocked artery by way of primary angioplasty or thrombolytic therapy. The patient needs to be treated with aspirin, clopidogrel, beta-blocker, ACE-inhibitor and anticoagulation with heparin. Morphine can be given to address the pain and anxiety.

BRUGADA SYNDROME

Brugada syndrome is a genetic disorder that can lead to sudden cardiac death due to ventricular fibrillation. This disorder may have characteristic ECG changes as described below. These changes involve ST segment elevation, together with incomplete RBBB pattern. While this is not so common among Caucasian populations, it is the most common cause of sudden cardiac death for young individuals in South East Asia and East Asia. The ECG changes are observed in the precordial leads, in particular in V_1, V_2 and V_3. Diagnosis is supported by a history of VF or VT, syncope or a family history of sudden cardiac death at a young age. Three types of ECG changes have been described.

Type 1

- ST segment elevation of about 2 mm with a gradual descent (the J point elevation is 2 mm or more), as shown in Figure 2.17
- ST segment elevation is convex upward (coved type)
- T wave inversion.

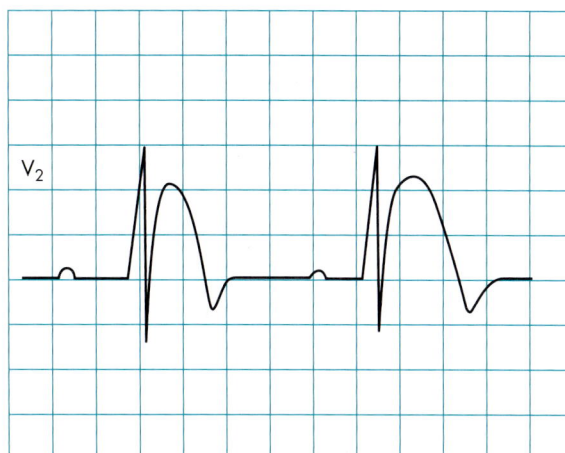

Figure 2.17 Brugada syndrome, type I

Type 2

- ST segment elevation of 1–2 mm (the J point is elevated 2 mm then the ST segment settles to 1 mm)
- ST segment elevation is concave upward (saddleback type)
- T waves are upright or biphasic.

Type 3

- ST segment elevation is less than 2 mm
- T wave is upright.

ST segment depression

ST segment depression could be due to multiple reasons. Morphologically, it could be horizontal, or sloping down or up. If the changes are dynamic in the right clinical context, it is clinically significant and warrants urgent remedial action. Some of the causes of ST segment depression are:

1 Pseudo ST segment depression is seen in sinus tachycardia as a J point depression or a junctional point depression, which is a normal variant
2 Hyperventilation
3 Effect of digoxin
4 Right ventricular hypertrophy or left ventricular hypertrophy — ST segment depression in this situation is seen in the corresponding ECG leads. It may also be associated with secondary ECG changes in left bundle branch block or right bundle branch block
5 Mitral valve prolapse

6   Acute coronary ischaemia — ST segment depression associated with coronary ischaemia presents with angina in a patient with coronary risk factors. Persistent ST segment depression with chest pain at rest could be unstable angina. Persistent ST segment depression with chest pain and positive biomarkers of cardiac injury, such as troponin, indicate acute subendocardial myocardial infarction

7   ST segment depression that is down sloping or horizontal during exercise stress testing may indicate underlying coronary artery stenosis

8   Diffuse and widespread ST segment depression with ST segment elevation in aVR is seen in the setting of significant stenosis or occlusion in the left main coronary artery. There can also be associated ST segment elevation in the lead V_1.

CLINICAL NOTES ON ST SEGMENT DEPRESSION DUE TO CORONARY ISCHAEMIA

If there is diagnostic ST segment depression observed in an exercise stress test, the patient needs to be referred for coronary angiography.

If ST segment depression is associated with angina at rest, the diagnosis is likely to be acute coronary syndrome. The management in this instance should include aspirin, clopidogrel, beta-blocker, ACE-inhibitor, statin therapy and anticoagulation with heparin. The patient may benefit from cardiac catheterisation.

T wave

The T wave is usually upright in leads I, II, V_3, V_4, V_5 and V_6. It is normally inverted in lead aVR and lead V_1. In lead III it can take the direction of the QRS complex.

T wave inversion can indicate coronary ischaemia or digitalis effect.

Wellens syndrome

This is a presentation of unstable angina due to a high-grade, critical stenosis of the proximal left anterior descending (LAD) artery with characteristic ECG changes. If not reopened early, this coronary stenosis can lead to a significant myocardial infarction involving the territory supplied by the LAD artery, the anteroseptal region of the left ventricle. ECG features (Fig 2.18) observed in Wellens syndrome include:

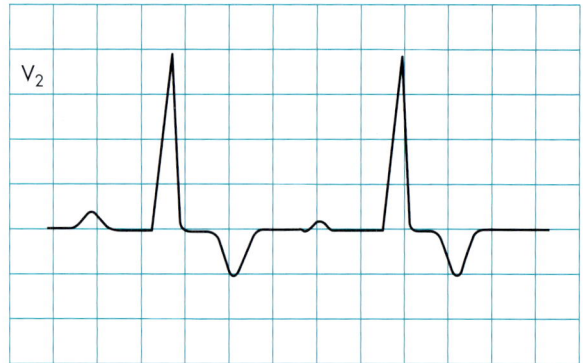

Figure 2.18 Wellens syndrome

- Deep T wave inversion in leads V_1 to V_4 and occasionally in V_5 and V_6 (sometimes deep T wave inversion could be limited to only V_2 and V_3). The sloping angle of the inverted T wave is 60°–90° and symmetrical

- Less commonly, instead of deep inversion the T wave may appear biphasic in V_3–V_5

- Precordial R wave progression is normal

- ST segments remain isoelectric or mildly elevated (by about 1 mm).

The patient may not show any elevation of cardiac biomarkers, such as troponin. However these patients need to be promptly stabilised with anticoagulant (heparin or enoxaparin) and anti-platelet (aspirin or clopidogrel) therapy and referred for coronary angiography. Often they require stent insertion to the proximal LAD segment.

U wave

The U wave comes immediately after the T wave and usually it is not seen in the standard ECG. It is smaller than one-third the height of the preceding T wave. It takes the same direction as the preceding T wave.

Prominent or large U waves are seen in:

- Hypokalaemia
- Hyperkalaemia
- Thyrotoxicosis
- Intracranial bleeding
- Long QT syndrome.

J wave (Osborn wave)

This is a smaller R wave seen immediately after the QRS complex and due to the elevation of the J point. The J wave is seen in:

- Hypothermia
- Hypocalcaemia.

OTHER PATHOLOGIES WITH MIXED ECG CHANGES

There are several cardiac and non-cardiac pathologies that can cause ECG changes. These changes are observed in different segments of the ECG complex, as discussed below.

Pulmonary embolism (PE)

ECG changes are rather insensitive in the diagnosis of acute pulmonary embolism. More commonly associated with PE are:

- Tachycardia (sinus or fast AF)
- Right axis deviation
- RBBB pattern indicating RV strain
- Non-specific ST segment shift or T wave inversions (T wave inversions are mostly seen in V_1 to V_3)
- An S1Q3T3 pattern that includes prominent S waves in lead I together with Q wave and T wave inversion in lead III
- The classic S1Q3T3 pattern is seen in only less than 15 per cent of cases with PE.

Subarachnoid haemorrhage (SAH)

ECG changes are seen in 50 per cent of SAH cases. These changes include:

- Prolonged QT interval
- Deep T wave inversion or tall positively oriented T waves
- ST segment depression or elevation
- Appearance of U waves.

Takotsubo cardiomyopathy

ECG changes of Takotsubo cardiomyopathy mimic that of anterior wall ST segment elevation myocardial infarction. Note there is ST segment elevation in leads V_2 to V_4 and occasionally V_5 and V_6. In the acute setting, there is ST segment elevation followed by deep T wave inversion together with prolongation of the QT interval. This phase can last for several days. In the next phase, the QT interval settles and the T wave inversion persists but at a smaller size. Takotsubo cardiomyopathy can present with new LBBB patterns too. The clinical picture could be either ischaemic chest pain or pulmonary oedema.

Hypokalaemia

Patients with very low serum potassium levels may have different ECG changes as described below. In addition, supraventricular tachyarrhythmias, ventricular tachycardia and ventricular fibrillation can be seen in this setting. Typical ECG manifestations of hypokalaemia include:

- T wave inversion
- ST segment depression
- Appearance of U waves
- Prolonged PR interval
- Prolonged QT interval.

Hypokalaemia is caused by aggressive diuretic therapy, diarrhoea or vomiting. Hypokalaemia is managed with intravenous or oral potassium replacement.

Hyperkalaemia

Hyperkalaemia is diagnosed when the serum potassium (K^+) level goes above 5.5 millimoles per litre. Above 6.0 millimoles per litre, it is considered moderate hyperkalaemia, and above 7.0 millimoles per litre, it is severe and places the patient at risk of cardiac arrest. The ECG changes (Fig 2.19) seen as the K^+ level rises are:

- Smaller P waves
- Tall T waves (tenting of T waves)
- Short QT interval
- ST segment depression.

These changes may progress to the following as the serum potassium level rises further:

- Prolongation of the QRS complex (bundle branch block pattern)
- Prolonged PR interval.

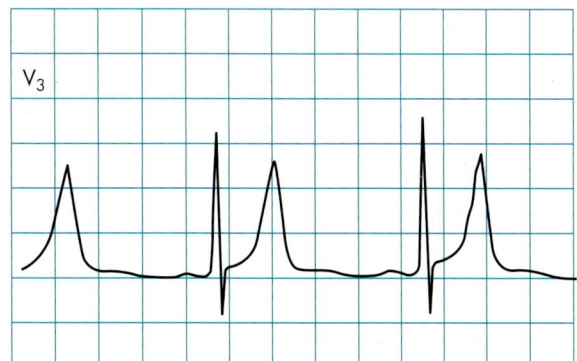

Figure 2.19 Hyperkalaemia

Further elevation of potassium levels will cause extreme widening of the QRS complex to resemble that of a sinusoidal wave form, which will degenerate rapidly into VT or asystole.

Hyperkalaemia is caused by severe renal failure, excess potassium replacement, ACE-inhibitor therapy, spironolactone and/or severe acidosis. When hyperkalaemia presents with ECG changes, it should be urgently managed with an intravenous infusion of $CaCl_2$ (calcium chloride). In addition, an infusion of insulin and dextrose should be commenced. Oral or per rectal resonium is given to remove excess potassium from the body. In severe renal failure, hyperkalaemia is an indication for dialysis. The cause of hyperkalaemia should be identified and corrected.

Digoxin toxicity

Digoxin at therapeutic (non-toxic) levels can bring about ST segment depression and T wave inversion on the ECG. However, in digoxin toxicity additional ECG changes (Fig 2.20) are observed including:

- Prolongation of the PR interval
- Progression to severe bradycardia with advanced heart block
- More prominent ST segment depression
- More prominent T wave inversion with a classic 'reverse tick' shape
- Shortening of the QT interval
- Ventricular ectopy or bigeminy
- Ventricular tachycardia progressing to ventricular fibrillation.

Tricyclic antidepressant overdose

A tricyclic antidepressant overdose can give rise to ECG changes. These changes are not too specific, but commonly seen changes include:

- Sinus tachycardia
- Prolongation of the PR interval
- Widening of the QRS complex
- Prolongation of the QT interval.

PACEMAKER

Pacemaker insertion is indicated when the intrinsic cardiac rhythm is unable to provide an adequate rate for the preservation of haemodynamic stability. Pacemaker activity on the ECG is signified by a short vertical line, called the 'pacemaker spike', that appears before the cardiac wave concerned (Fig 2.21).

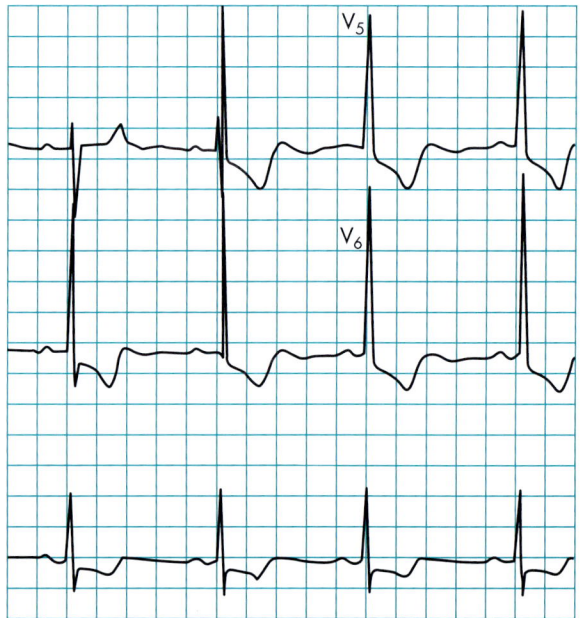

Figure 2.20 Digoxin toxicity with 'reverse tick' T wave inversion

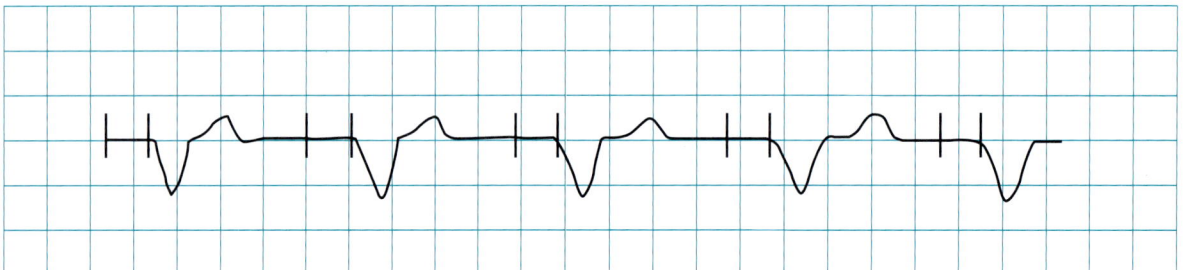

Figure 2.21 AV paced rhythm (atrial and ventricular pacing spikes)

If the right atrium is paced the spike appears just before the P wave, and if the ventricle is paced it appears just before the QRS complex. If both the atrium and the ventricle are paced—called dual chamber pacing—you see two spikes, one before the P wave and the other before the QRS complex.

If the sinus activity is preserved and the pacemaker is inserted due to AV nodal disease or conduction defect below the AV node, the pacemaker can be programmed to sense the sinus or atrial activity. Thus the ventricular impulse can be delivered to complement the atrial activity. This is called atrial (A) sensed ventricular (V) pacing.

REFERENCES

1 Brugada P, Brugada J, Mont L, Smeets J 1991 A new approach to the differential diagnosis of a regular tachycardia with a wide QRS complex. Circulation 83:1649–1659

2 Garmel G M 2008 Wide complex tachycardias: understanding this complex condition: Part 1 Epidemiology and electrophysiology. Western J Emergency Medicine Jan 9(1):28–39

3 Kindwall K E, Brown J, Josephson M E 1988 Electrocardiographic criteria for ventricular tachycardia in wide-complex left bundle branch morphology tachycardias. American J Cardiology 61:1279–1283

ECGS AND PATHOLOGIES

Instructions on the ECG worksheets

This section of this workbook contains a series of ECG tracings with a brief introductory clinical vignette. The ECG worksheet is provided to guide the reader to approach ECG interpretation in a systematic manner. The worksheet is repeated for each ECG so as to facilitate repetitive learning. This is the optimal way to practise the systematic approach to ECG reading.

Each case accompanies an answer sheet that provides information on the significant changes observed on the ECG and a brief note on management based on the most likely diagnosis. The reader may notice when filling in the worksheet that some parameters fall within the normal limits of measurement as per the information provided in previous sections of this workbook. The normal parameters are not always included in the answer so as to concentrate the focus on the salient abnormalities and also to maintain brevity and clarity.

Please note that this workbook is not a therapeutic manual. It is an aid for the junior clinician to learn and practise how to read ECG in a systematic manner. The clinical notes including those related to physical examination, investigations and management are aimed at helping the clinician to develop the ability to interpret ECGs in the right clinical context, as is the case in real-life practice. Thus these notes are kept concise to fulfil the task of training the reader to think in a logical manner, maintaining the focus on the 'whole patient' when reading an ECG in the clinical setting. All ECGs are obtained from real patients in a clinical practice. Some ECGs have multiple abnormalities as in real-life situations. The ECGs are arranged randomly, again to mirror the clinical setting.

The first ECG is normal. The worksheet following this ECG is answered verbatim as an example to the reader on how to proceed through the rest of the worksheets. The subsequent answers contain only the important abnormalities and clinical information that would help the reader with self-assessment.

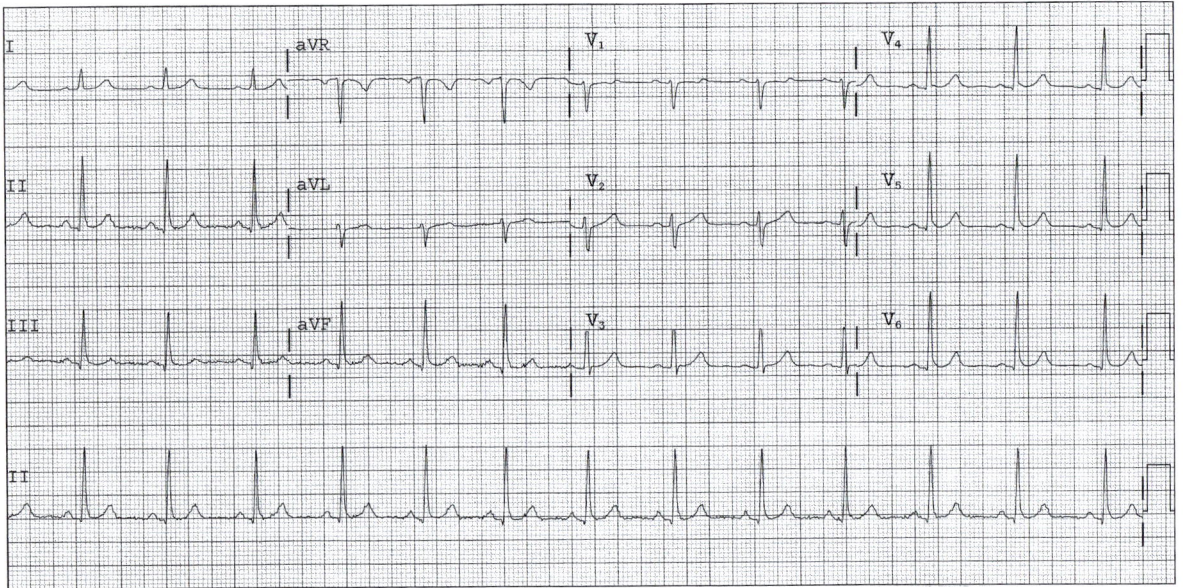

Figure 3.1a

CASE STUDY ON ECG 1

Please interpret the ECG in Figure 3.1a in a systematic manner.

Rhythm _____

Rate _____

Axis _____

P wave _____

PR interval _____

QRS complex _____

ST segment _____

T wave morphology _____

QT interval _____

Conclusion _____

Clinical notes _____

Diagnosis _____

_____

_____

_____

_____

Further investigations _____

_____

_____

_____

Management _____

_____

_____

_____

_____

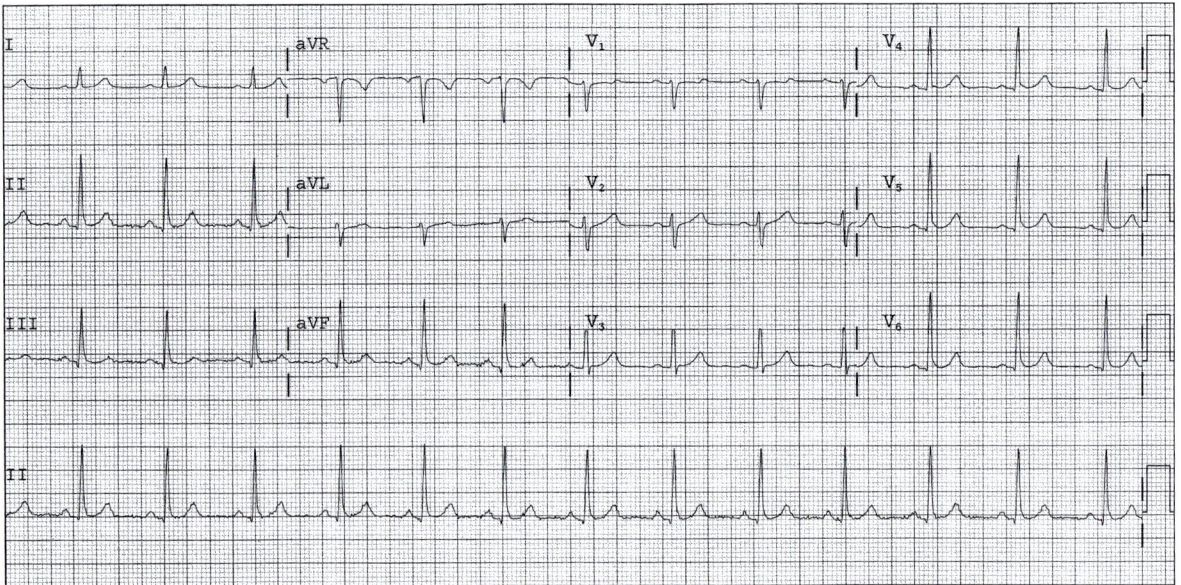

Figure 3.1b Normal ECG

ANSWER TO CASE STUDY ON ECG 1: NORMAL ECG

Refer to Figure 3.1b.

Rhythm Sinus

Rate 80 bpm

Axis 71° and normal

P wave Normal size and morphology

PR interval 162 ms and normal

QRS complex Normal morphology, amplitude and width. QRS complex is 90 ms wide.

T wave morphology Normal size and morphology. Upright in all leads.

ST segment Remains at baseline.

QT interval Normal at 411 ms

Conclusion This ECG is normal so it does not indicate any underlying cardiac pathology.

Clinical notes Normal ECG parameters and waveforms

Diagnosis No evident cardiac pathology

Further investigations None required

Management None indicated

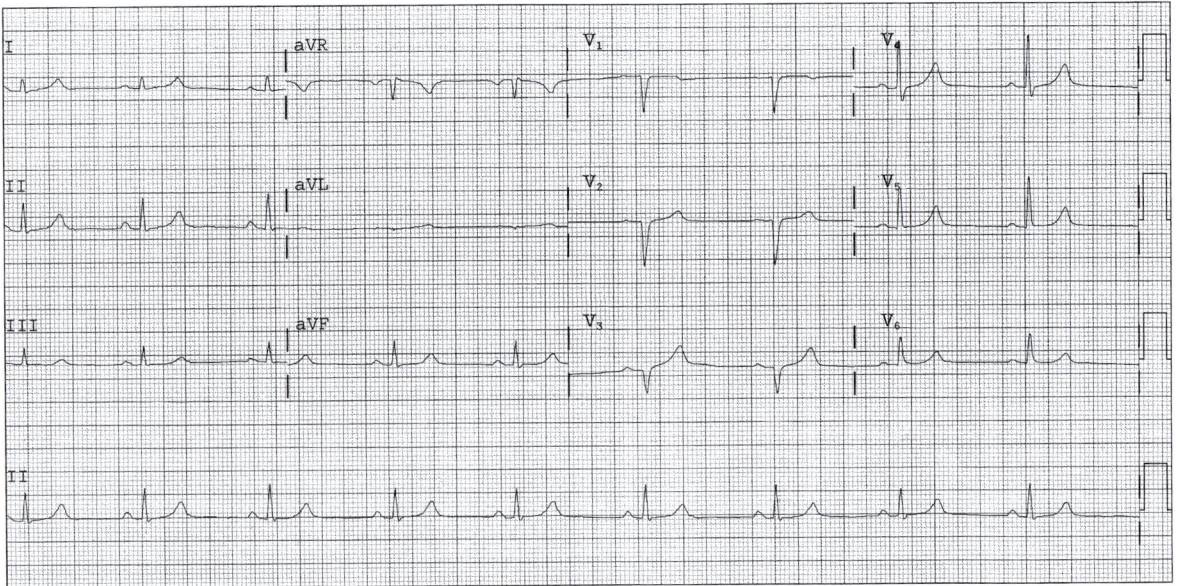

Figure 3.2a

CASE STUDY ON ECG 2

A 57-year-old man presents with progressive dyspnoea, orthopnoea and paroxysmal nocturnal dyspnoea, together with progressive ankle oedema. He has a background history of chronic diabetes, hypertension and hypercholesterolaemia. Upon further assessment an ECG was obtained.

Please interpret the ECG in Figure 3.2a in a systematic manner.

Rhythm _____

Rate _____

Axis _____

P wave _____

PR interval _____

QRS complex _____

ST segment _____

T wave morphology _____

QT interval _____

Conclusion _____

Clinical notes _____

Diagnosis _____

_____

_____

_____

_____

Further investigations _____

_____

_____

_____

_____

Management _____

_____

_____

_____

_____

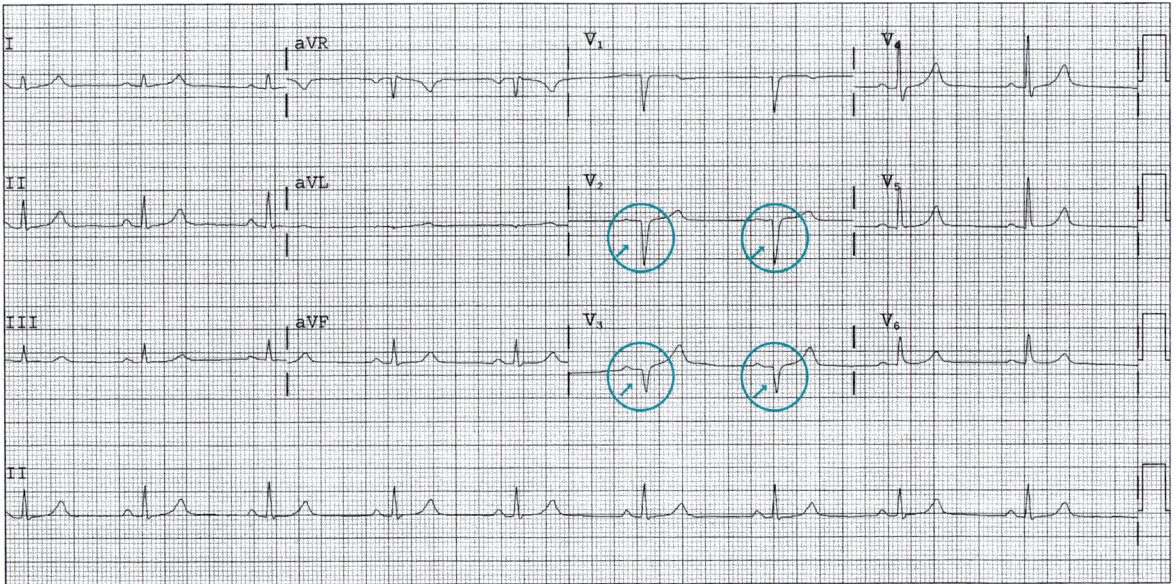

Figure 3.2b Sinus rhythm and septal Q waves

ANSWER TO CASE STUDY ON ECG 2: SINUS RHYTHM AND SEPTAL Q WAVES

A

The rhythm is regular, the rate is 54 bpm and the axis is within normal limits (Fig 3.2b).

The important abnormalities seen in the ECG are the Q waves in the anterior leads V_1, V_2 and V_3 (shown by arrows) suggesting previous myocardial infarction. However there is no past history to this effect. Given his diabetes, it is possible that the patient may have had a silent myocardial infarction in the past. The current presentation is likely to be due to ischaemic systolic heart failure. Hypertension too can contribute to heart failure. Diabetes can give rise to diastolic heart failure.

In the physical examination look for signs of heart failure, such as elevated jugular venous pressure (JVP), S3 gallop, pulmonary crepitations and peripheral oedema. Describe the severity of his condition according to the NYHA functional class (see Appendix). Given that he has symptoms at rest, he belongs to NYHA class IV.

In addition to the ECG he needs a full blood count, electrolyte profile, cardiac biomarkers (troponin T or I) and his renal function indices checked. He needs a chest X-ray to look for pulmonary congestion and an echocardiogram to evaluate his left ventricular function.

Once the diagnosis of heart failure is confirmed, he needs to be treated with diuretics and nitrates to relieve congestion. If his left ventricular ejection fraction is less than 40 per cent, he may require fluid restriction to 1.0–1.5 L per day. He needs to be weighed daily to monitor significant and rapid weight gain that would suggest fluid overload. He needs to be treated with an ACE inhibitor if the blood pressure is satisfactory. He needs to be commenced on a beta-blocker when he is compensated. His coronary risk factors need to be well controlled. If there is evidence of acute coronary ischaemia in the way of dynamic ECG changes or positive biomarkers, he needs to be referred for coronary angiography.

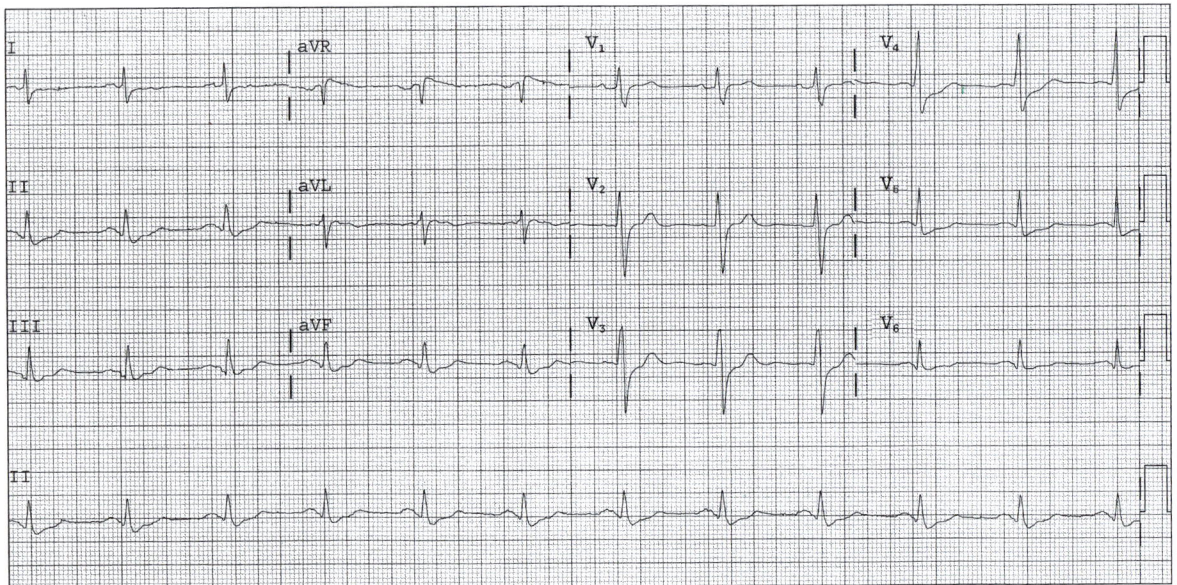

Figure 3.3a

CASE STUDY ON ECG 3

A 64-year-old man presents with retrosternal chest tightness at rest. The sublingual nitrates administered by the paramedics relieved the chest pain. He has a background history of hypertension and smoking. Upon further assessment an ECG was obtained.

Please interpret the ECG in Figure 3.3a in a systematic manner.

Rhythm _____

Rate _____

Axis _____

P wave _____

PR interval _____

QRS complex _____

ST segment _____

T wave morphology _____

QT interval _____

Conclusion _____

Clinical notes _____

Diagnosis _____

_____

_____

_____

_____

Further investigations _____

_____

_____

_____

_____

Management _____

_____

_____

_____

_____

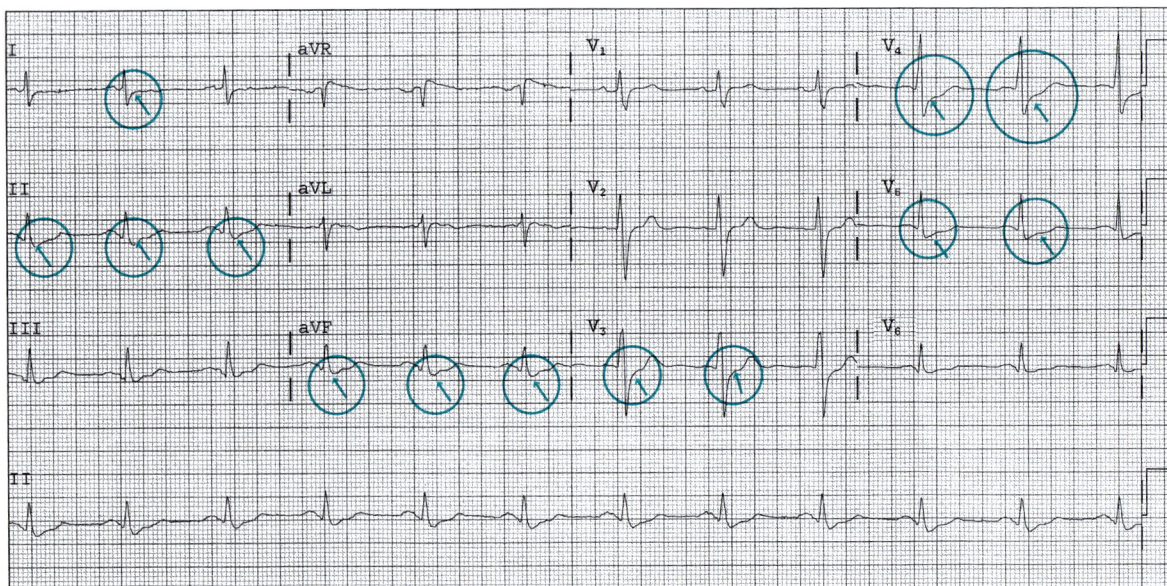

Figure 3.3b Non ST elevation acute coronary syndrome

ANSWER TO CASE STUDY ON ECG 3: NON ST ELEVATION ACUTE CORONARY SYNDROME

A

This man is in sinus rhythm. His heart rate is 68 bpm. The axis is more towards the right (90°). The QRS complex is 120 ms, just at the upper limit of the normal range (Fig 3.3b).

The most important observation is the ST segment depression seen in leads II, aVF, V_3, V_4 and V_5 and shown by arrows. This is called 'widespread' ST segment depression. In the light of his symptoms and risk factors these ECG changes are highly suggestive of severe global coronary ischaemia. He needs to be stabilised by the administration of antiplatelet therapy in the way of aspirin and clopidogrel. He will benefit from nitrates (given intravenously, orally or topically) and morphine for symptom-relief. He should be anticoagulated with intravenous heparin or subcutaneous unfractionated heparin. He also needs treatment with ACE inhibitor, beta-blocker and a statin.

His cardiac biomarkers should be checked.

He may benefit from early catheterisation, especially if the cardiac biomarkers are elevated.

He needs to be admitted to the coronary care unit for cardiac monitoring. His risk factors need to be aggressively controlled.

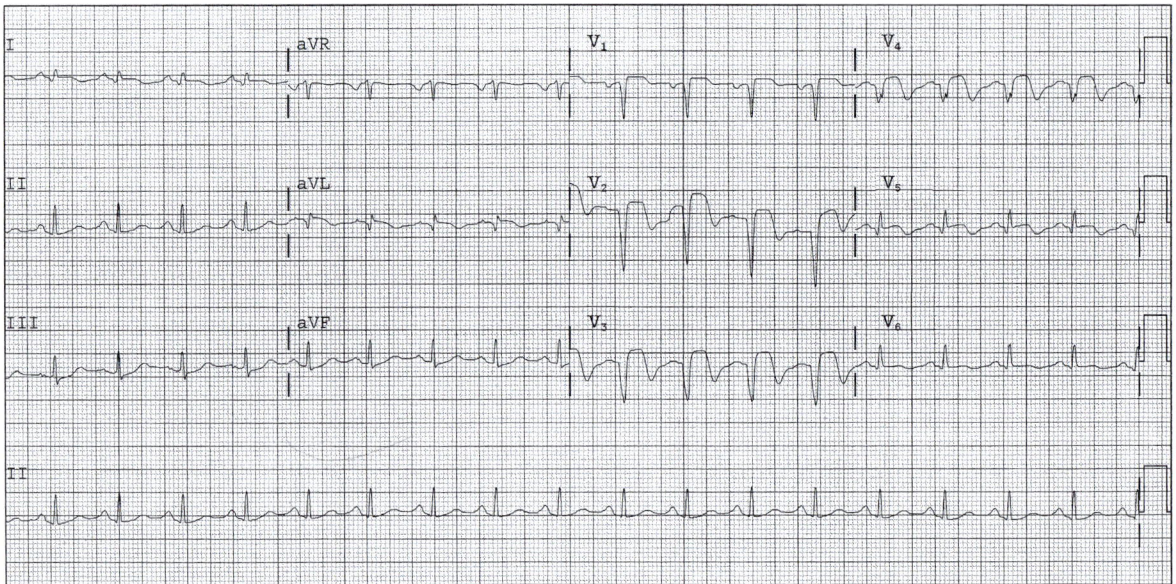

Figure 3.4a

CASE STUDY ON ECG 4

This 64-year-old man presents with severe retrosternal chest pain of 3 hours' duration. He was diaphoretic at presentation. He has a positive family history for ischaemic heart disease. Upon further assessment an ECG was obtained.

Please interpret the ECG in Figure 3.4a in a systematic manner.

Rhythm _____

Rate _____

Axis _____

P wave _____

PR interval _____

QRS complex _____

ST segment _____

T wave morphology _____

QT interval _____

Conclusion _____

Clinical notes _____

Diagnosis _____

_____

_____

_____

_____

Further investigations _____

_____

_____

_____

_____

Management _____

_____

_____

_____

_____

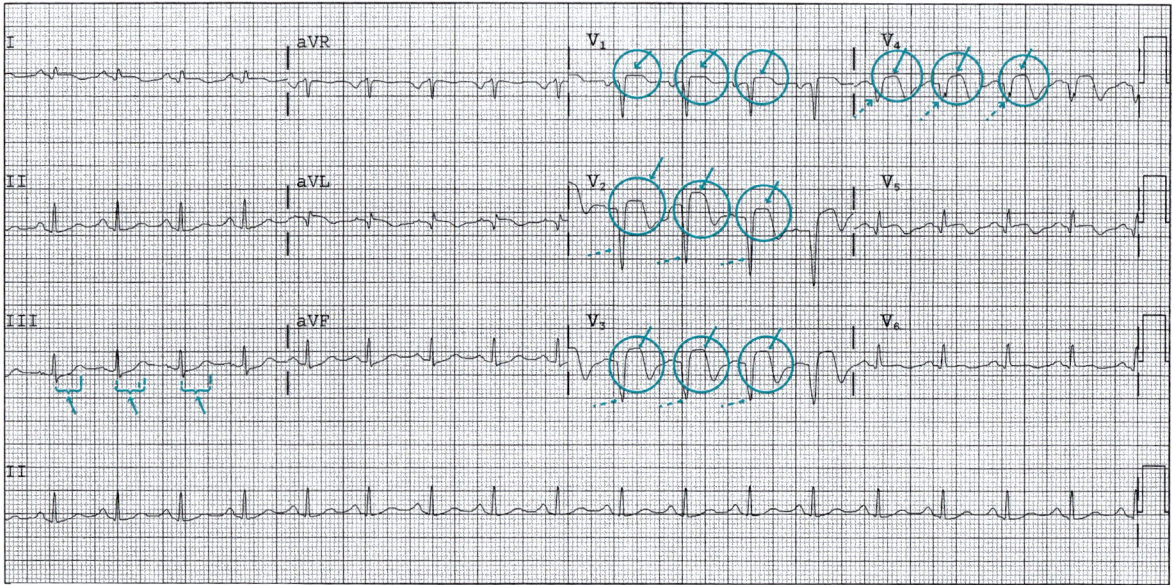

Figure 3.4b Anterior ST elevation infarction

ANSWER TO CASE STUDY ON ECG 4: ANTERIOR ST ELEVATION INFARCTION

A

This man is in sinus rhythm with tachycardia at a heart rate of 100 bpm. Axis is deviated to the right (Fig 3.4b).

The most important feature is the significant ST segment elevation seen in leads V_1, V_2, V_3 and V_4 (thin arrows). The leads V_2, V_3 and V_4 also have Q waves (dotted arrows). There is ST segment elevation also in leads I and aVL. This is anterolateral ST segment elevation myocardial infarction (STEMI).

The QT interval is prolonged. The QT prolongation could be due to acute ischaemia. He needs to be stabilised with antiplatelet therapy, anticoagulants and oxygen via mask (particularly if he is de-saturating). Intravenous nitrates or morphine should be given for the chest pain provided that he is not severely hypotensive. Organise urgent reperfusion therapy with primary angioplasty if available or thrombolytic therapy if primary angioplasty facility is not readily available and if there is no contraindication.

This ECG and clinical vignette highlights the importance of rapid assessment and immediate ECG reading in the setting of chest pain that suggests coronary ischaemia.

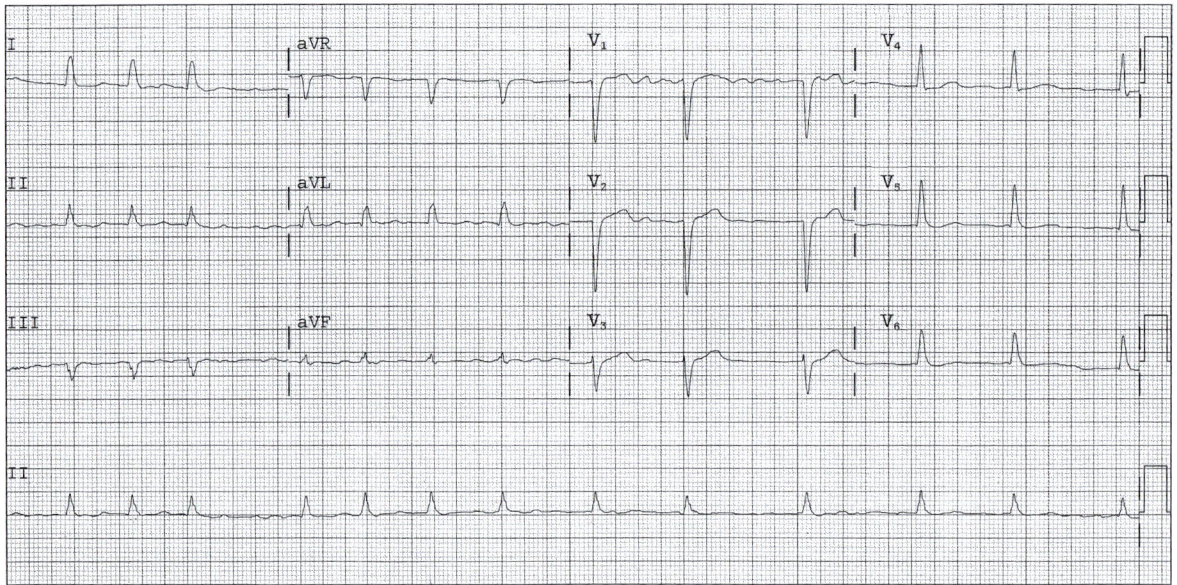

Figure 3.5a

CASE STUDY ON ECG 5

Q

A 75-year-old woman presents with palpitations and dyspnoea. She has a background history of hypertension, diabetes mellitus and congestive cardiac failure. She had a myocardial infarction nine years ago. Upon further assessment an ECG was obtained.

Please interpret the ECG in Figure 3.5a in a systematic manner.

Rhythm _____

Rate _____

Axis _____

P wave _____

PR interval _____

QRS complex _____

ST segment _____

T wave morphology _____

QT interval _____

Conclusion _____

Clinical notes _____

Diagnosis _____

_____

_____

_____

_____

Further investigations _____

_____

_____

_____

_____

Management _____

_____

_____

_____

_____

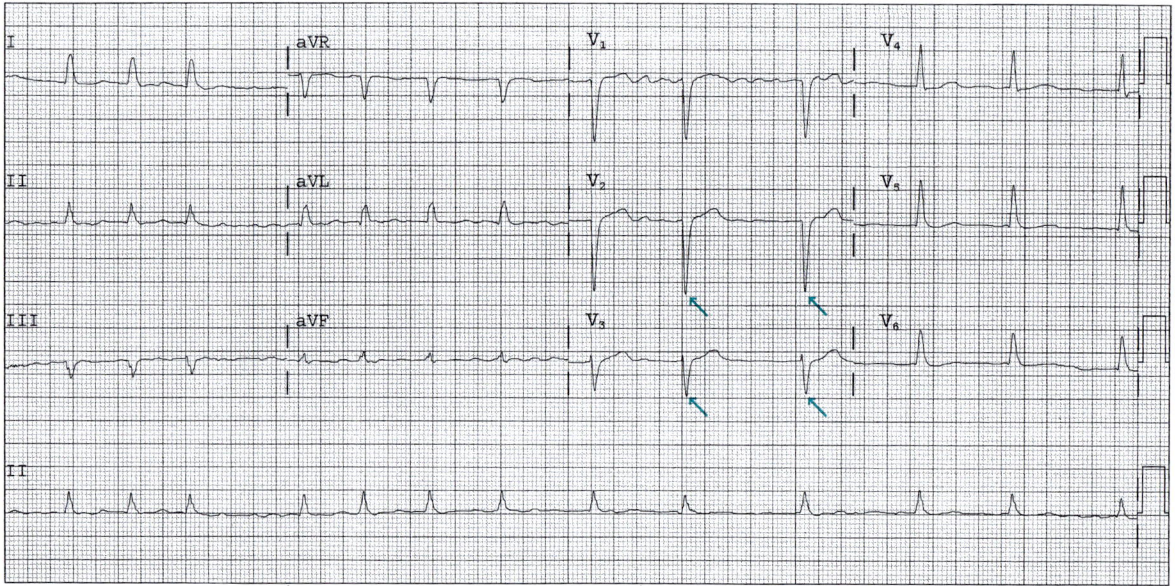

Figure 3.5b Atrial fibrillation

ANSWER TO CASE STUDY ON ECG 5: ATRIAL FIBRILLATION

A

Note that the rhythm is irregularly irregular (Fig 3.5b). The heart rate is well controlled currently at 75 bpm, possibly on a beta-blocker, digoxin or a non-dihydropyridine calcium channel blocker.

The Q waves in the anterior/septal leads (V$_2$, V$_3$) are significant and indicate previous myocardial infarction (arrows). This is consistent with her past history. The new-onset atrial fibrillation can lead to decompensated heart failure.

Ischaemic heart disease, heart failure and chronic hypertension can lead to the development of atrial fibrillation. Given her increased stroke risk with a CHADS2 score of 4 (diabetes, hypertension, heart failure and age of 75 years), the patient needs prophylactic anticoagulation with warfarin or dabigatran unless there is a contraindication.

Her heart rate is controlled, hence the patient does not need any further therapy for rate control. If she develops recurrent symptoms, cardioversion with DC current or an anti-arrhythmic agent should be considered.

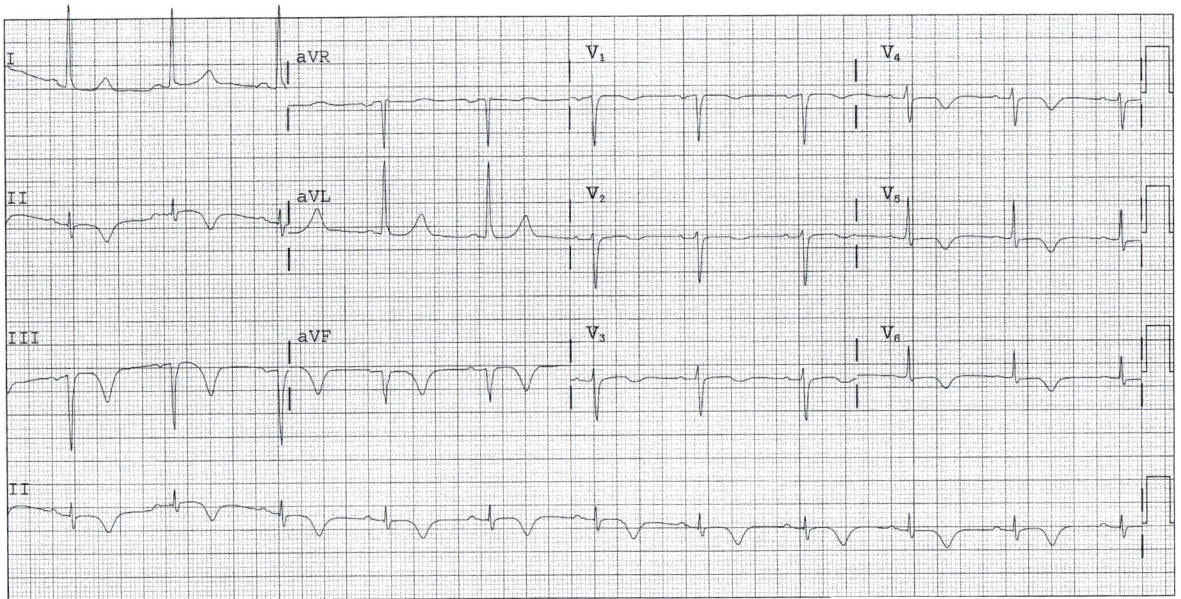

Figure 3.6a

CASE STUDY ON ECG 6

This 57-year-old man was assessed in the outpatient clinic for progressively worsening chest pain. He has a long-standing history of poorly controlled hypertension despite being treated with an ACE inhibitor. Upon further assessment an ECG was obtained.

Please interpret the ECG in Figure 3.6a in a systematic manner.

Rhythm _____

Rate _____

Axis _____

P wave _____

PR interval _____

QRS complex _____

ST segment _____

T wave morphology _____

QT interval _____

Conclusion _____

Clinical notes _____

Diagnosis _____

_____

_____

_____

_____

Further investigations _____

_____

_____

_____

_____

Management _____

_____

_____

_____

_____

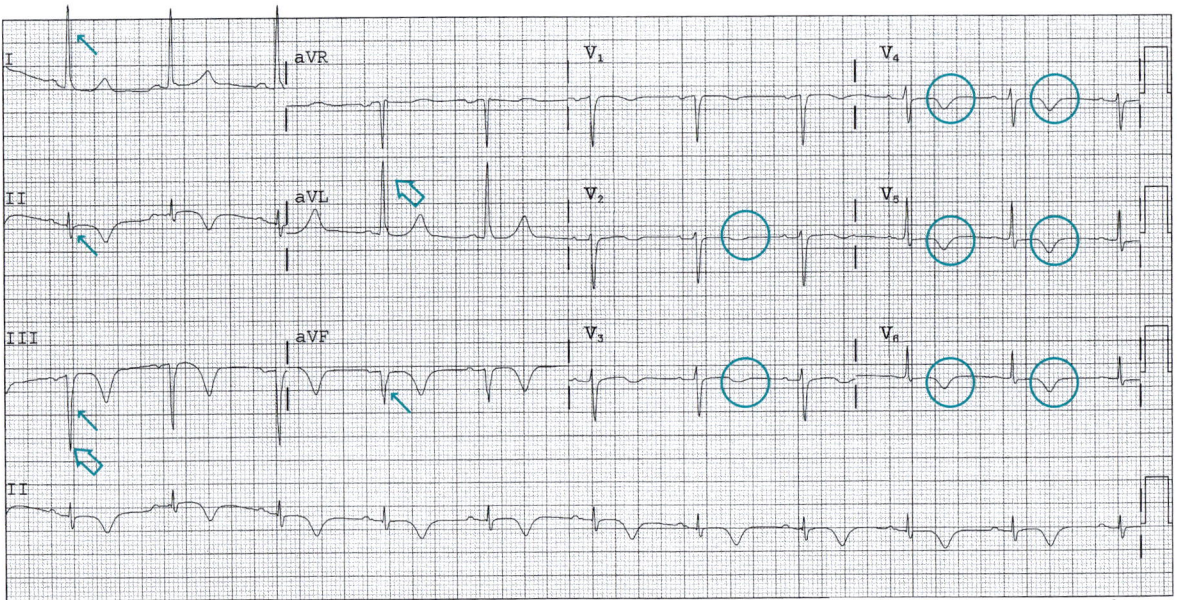

Figure 3.6b Left ventricular hypertrophy

ANSWER TO CASE STUDY ON ECG 6:
LEFT VENTRICULAR HYPERTROPHY

A

The rhythm is regular and the heart rate is 65 bpm (Fig 3.6b). Note the left axis deviation (LAD). Using the two-lead method you can see the QRS complex in lead I is predominantly upwardly deflected and that of aVF is downward (thin arrows). Using the three-lead method you can see that the QRS complex in lead I is predominantly positive (upwards) with that of leads II and III predominantly negative (downwards).

These changes can also be due to ischaemia in the inferior region of the left ventricle.

Left axis deviation together with tall R wave in lead aVL and deep S wave in lead III strongly suggest left ventricular hypertrophy (thick arrows).

T wave inversion seen in leads V_2, V_3, V_4, V_5 and V_6 (circles) can be due to left ventricular hypertrophy or coronary ischaemia. The T wave inversion in the inferior leads (leads II, III and aVF) together with the above similar changes in the anterolateral precordial or chest leads may also indicate diffuse coronary ischaemia affecting multiple vascular territories.

This patient needs an echocardiogram to confirm left ventricular hypertrophy and also to assess for any ischaemia. He needs to be admitted for further ECG monitoring and cardiac biomarker testing. He needs to be treated with anticoagulation and antiplatelet therapy.

His blood pressure needs to be controlled with dose increment of the ACE inhibitor or with the addition of another agent such as a dihydropyridine calcium channel blocker. The patient's coronary risk factors need detailed evaluation and aggressive control. To this effect his blood sugar level and cholesterol profile need to be checked and managed accordingly.

He may require further investigation for coronary ischaemia with coronary angiography.

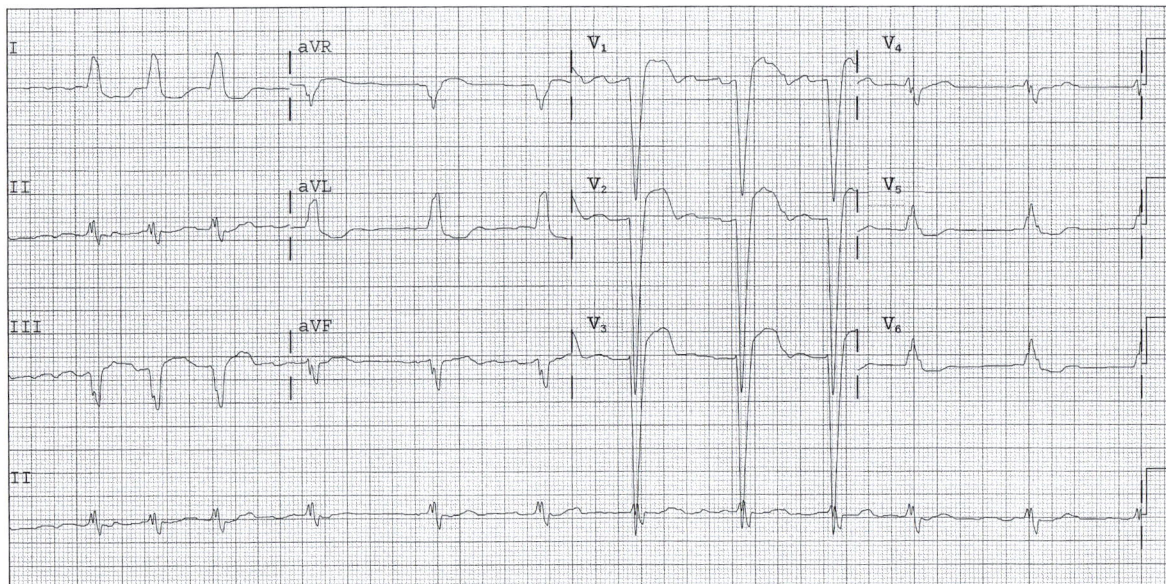

Figure 3.7a

CASE STUDY ON ECG 7

An 85-year-old woman presents with severe retrosternal and epigastric pain. She is otherwise well and very functional. She is independent. Upon further assessment an ECG was obtained. Previous clinical records indicate that the ECG changes noted in the current tracing are new. Importantly, there was no conduction defect seen in her old ECGs.

Please interpret the ECG in Figure 3.7a in a systematic manner.

Rhythm _____

Rate _____

Axis _____

P wave _____

PR interval _____

QRS complex _____

ST segment _____

T wave morphology _____

QT interval _____

Conclusion _____

Clinical notes _____

Diagnosis _____

_____

_____

_____

_____

Further investigations _____

_____

_____

_____

_____

Management _____

_____

_____

_____

_____

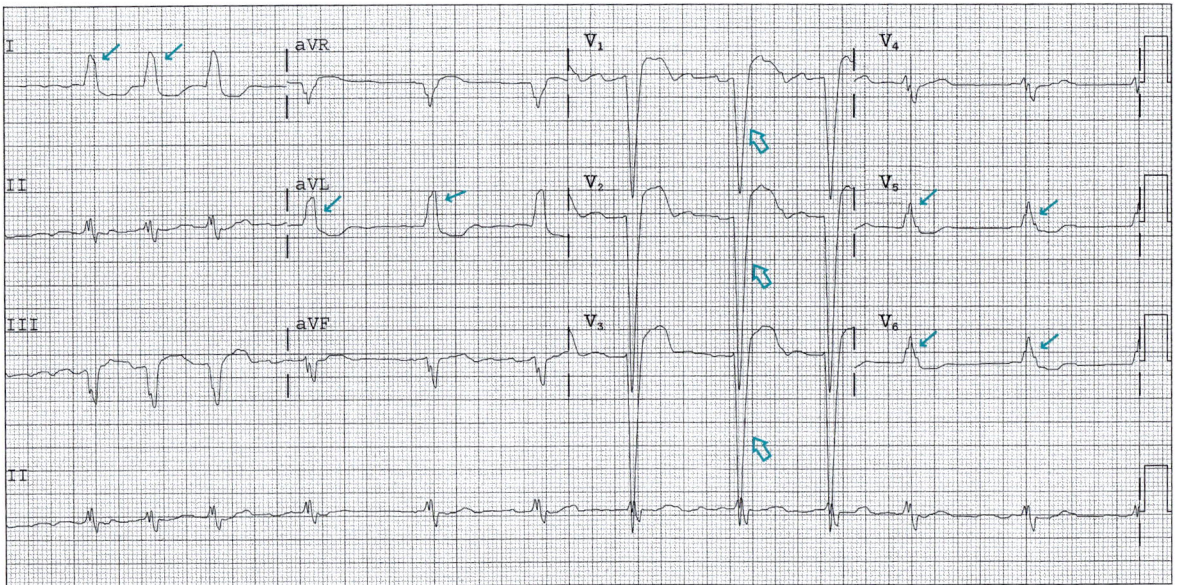

Figure 3.7b Left bundle branch block

ANSWER TO CASE STUDY ON ECG 7: LEFT BUNDLE BRANCH BLOCK

A

Note that the rhythm is irregularly irregular, hence atrial fibrillation. The rate is approximately 80 bpm (Fig 3.7b). The axis is deviated to the left (LAD).

The QRS complex is broad (duration of 158 ms). Note the features of LBBB:

- LAD with wide QRS complex of more than 120 ms
- Prominent and wide R waves are seen in leads V_5, V_6, aVL and I (thin arrows)
- Prominent S wave or QS complex is in leads V_1, V_2 and V_3 (thick arrows).

There is poor R wave progression in leads V_1 to V_3.

Usually ST segment depression or T wave inversion is seen as a feature of LBBB. In LBBB, ST segment is depressed in V_5 and V_6 and elevated in V_1, V_2 and V_3.

The ST segment shift secondary to LBBB is always in the opposite direction to that of the QRS complex. This phenomenon is called 'discordant ST segment shift due to the bundle branch block'.

When the ST segment shift is *concordant*, it is specifically indicative of acute myocardial infarction (hence the memory cue 'Con-In': concordant-infarction).

So, in this woman the significant ST segment elevation that is *discordant* to the QRS complex in leads V_1, V_2 and V_3 could be a secondary change due to the LBBB. However ST segment elevation secondary to LBBB has a concave-up morphology. The convex-up morphology in this case may perhaps indicate an anteroseptal acute infarct.

From a comparison with the patient's prior ECG records on previous non-cardiac admissions it was evident that the LBBB is new. The presence of a new LBBB with chest pain is highly likely to be due to acute myocardial infarction.

She needs to be stabilised with antiplatelet therapy, anticoagulants, intravenous morphine and glyceryl trinitrate therapy. She should be referred to the cardiac catheterisation laboratory for urgent catheterisation. The likely angiographic finding is a completely occluded left anterior descending artery. This occluded artery requires reopening by primary angioplasty and treatment with stent implantation.

Once coronary stents are placed the patient may require long-term antiplatelet therapy. In addition, she runs a high risk of stroke due to AF. Hence she may require long-term anticoagulation for stroke prevention. The combination of antiplatelet therapy and anticoagulation can place her at high risk of bleeding. This is a clinical dilemma that needs cautious management.

This case highlights the importance of always comparing the current ECG with the previous ECGs (if available) to ascertain whether any change observed is new.

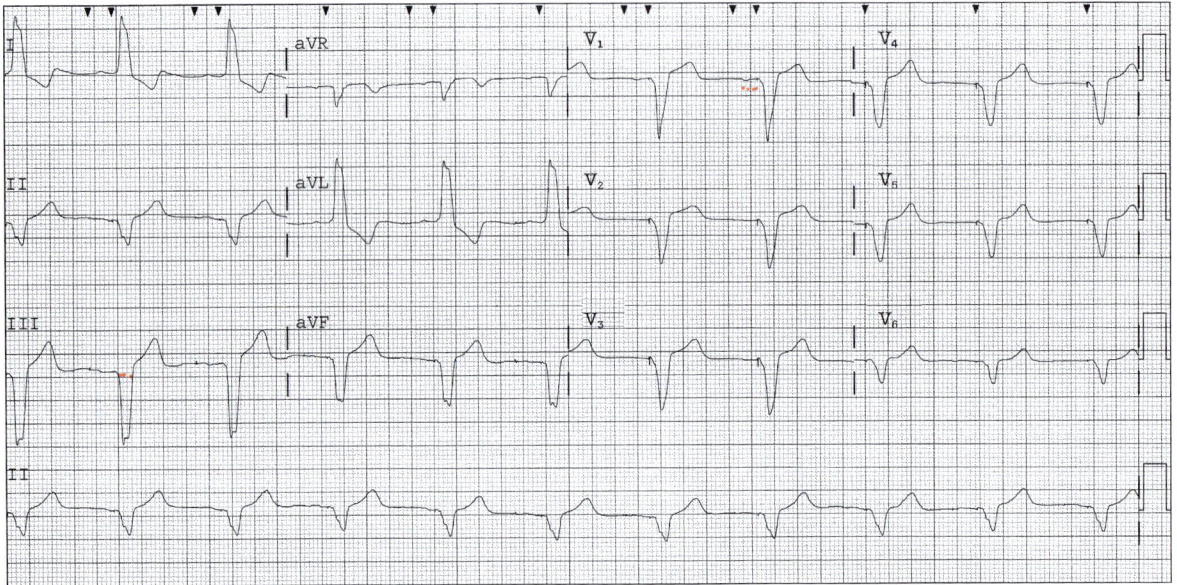

Figure 3.8a

CASE STUDY ON ECG 8

A 79-year-old man presents with syncope. Upon further assessment an ECG was obtained.

Please interpret the ECG in Figure 3.8a in a systematic manner.

Rhythm _____

Rate _____

Axis _____

P wave _____

PR interval _____

QRS complex _____

ST segment _____

T wave morphology _____

QT interval _____

Conclusion _____

Clinical notes _____

Diagnosis _____

_____

_____

_____

_____

Further investigations _____

_____

_____

_____

Management _____

_____

_____

_____

_____

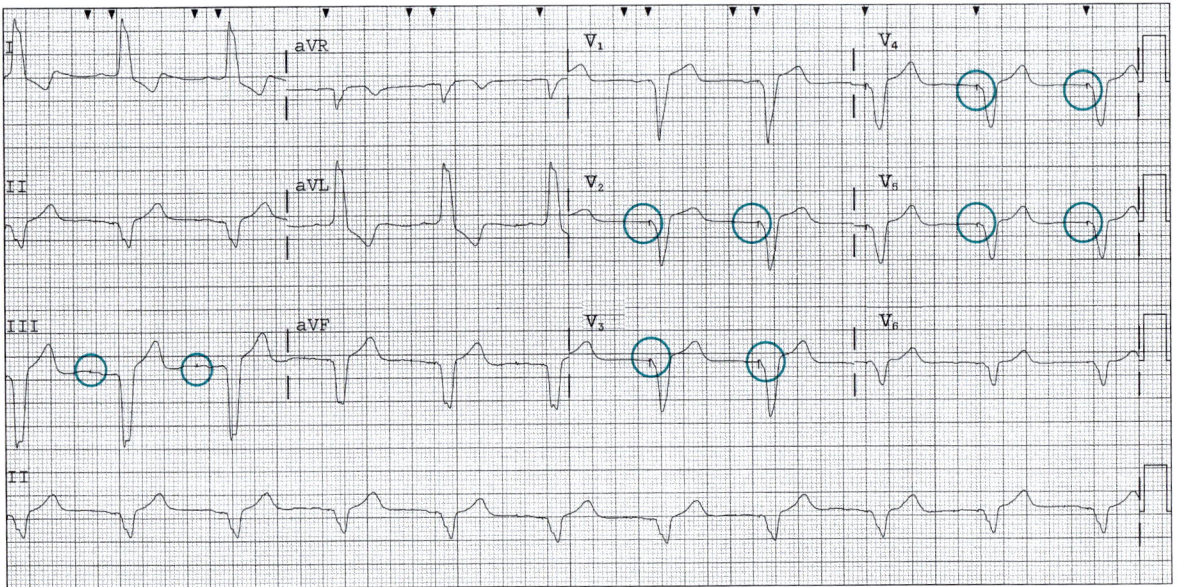

Figure 3.8b Paced rhythm

ANSWER TO CASE STUDY ON ECG 8: PACED RHYTHM

The rhythm is regular, the rate is 63 bpm and the axis is −50°, deviated to the left (Fig 3.8b).

Please note the paced rhythm on this ECG. The QRS complex is wide indicating the ventricular origin of the electrical impulse.

Pacing spikes seen as short vertical lines on the ECG indicate the presence of an implanted cardiac pacemaker. The atrial pacing spikes are seen as short vertical lines preceding each P wave, and ventricular pacing spikes precede the QRS complex (circles). The atrial pacing spikes are best seen in lead III and ventricular pacing spikes in leads V_2, V_3, V_4 and V_5.

It is important to exclude pacemaker malfunction as a cause for his syncope as he seems to be fully dependent on the pacemaker rhythm. This can be achieved by interrogating the pacemaker. Hence the patient should be referred to the cardiology team.

The other cardiovascular causes for syncope in this situation could include hypotension due to dehydration, antihypertensive agents or vasovagal attack. Remember that neurological pathologies, including epilepsy, and intracranial lesions can also cause syncope.

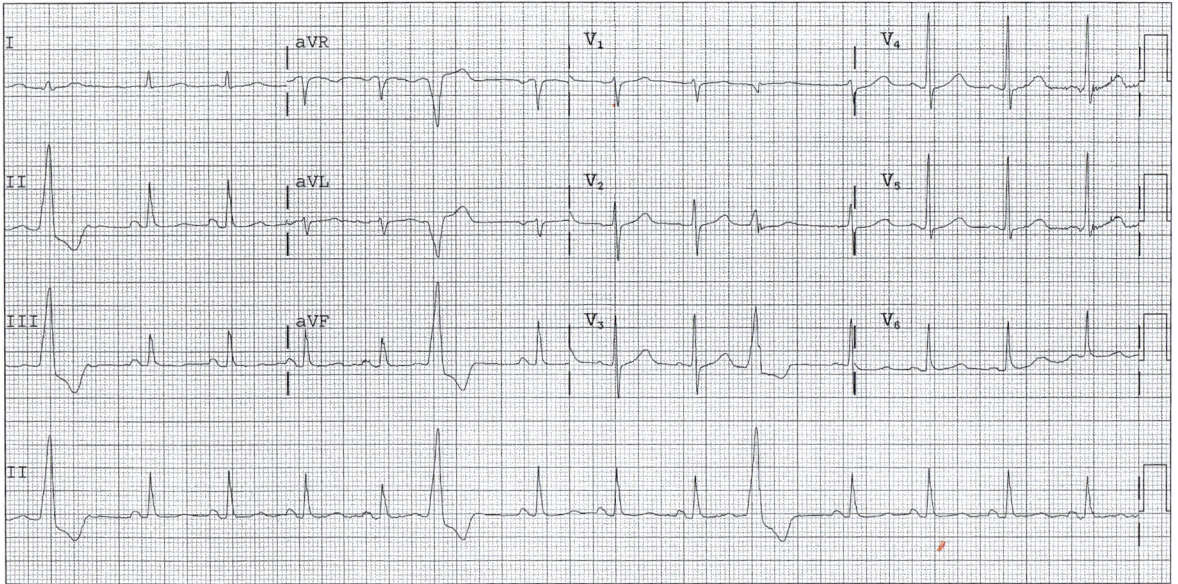

Figure 3.9a

CASE STUDY ON ECG 9

This 68-year-old man presents with palpitations and occasional exertion-related chest tightness. Upon further assessment an ECG was obtained.

Please interpret the ECG in Figure 3.9a in a systematic manner.

Rhythm _____

Rate _____

Axis _____

P wave _____

PR interval _____

QRS complex _____

ST segment _____

T wave morphology _____

QT interval _____

Conclusion _____

Clinical notes _____

Diagnosis _____

_____

_____

_____

_____

Further investigations _____

_____

_____

_____

Management _____

_____

_____

_____

_____

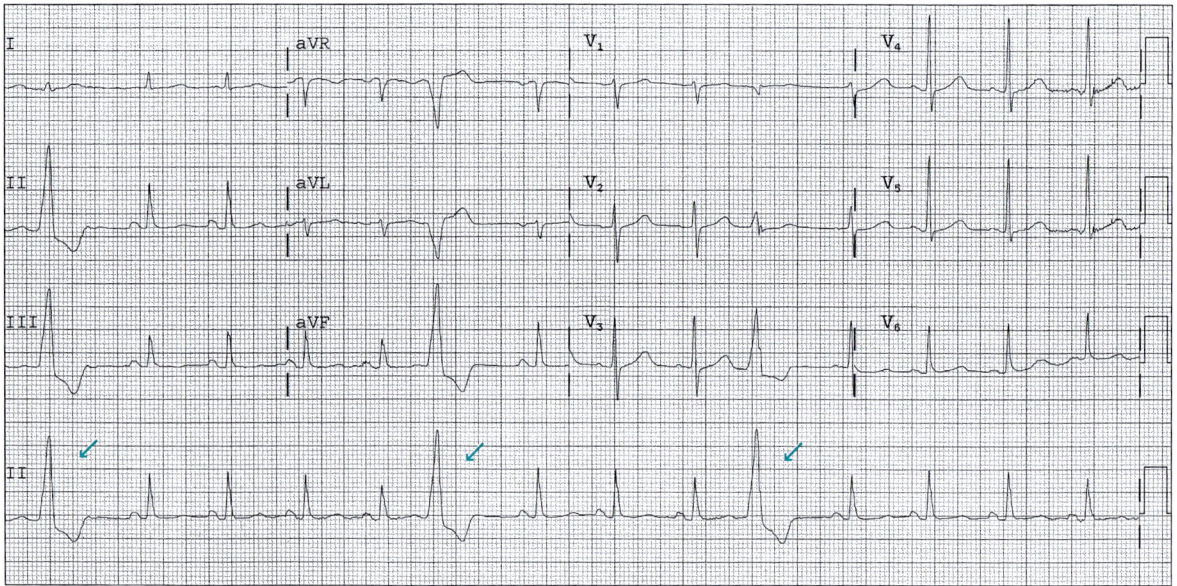

Figure 3.9b Ventricular ectopics

ANSWER TO CASE STUDY ON ECG 9: VENTRICULAR ECTOPICS

A

The rhythm is regular, the rate is 87 bpm and the axis is 80° (Fig 3.9b).

Note that the patient is in sinus rhythm. The QRS axis is in the normal direction.

The clinically relevant important observation to the patient's presenting complaint is the frequent occurrence of ventricular ectopic beats (VEBs) (arrows). These may contribute to the palpitations experienced by the patient, particularly if the VEBs are very frequent. In addition, note the prolonged QT interval. These two ECG changes together with the chest pain on exertion could suggest underlying ischaemic heart disease, hence the diagnosis of chronic stable angina.

The patient may benefit from further investigation with exercise stress test, exercise stress echocardiography or myocardial perfusion scan to evaluate for coronary ischaemia. If these non-invasive investigations for coronary ischaemia are positive, he needs referral for coronary angiography.

His coronary risk factors need to be assessed and managed accordingly.

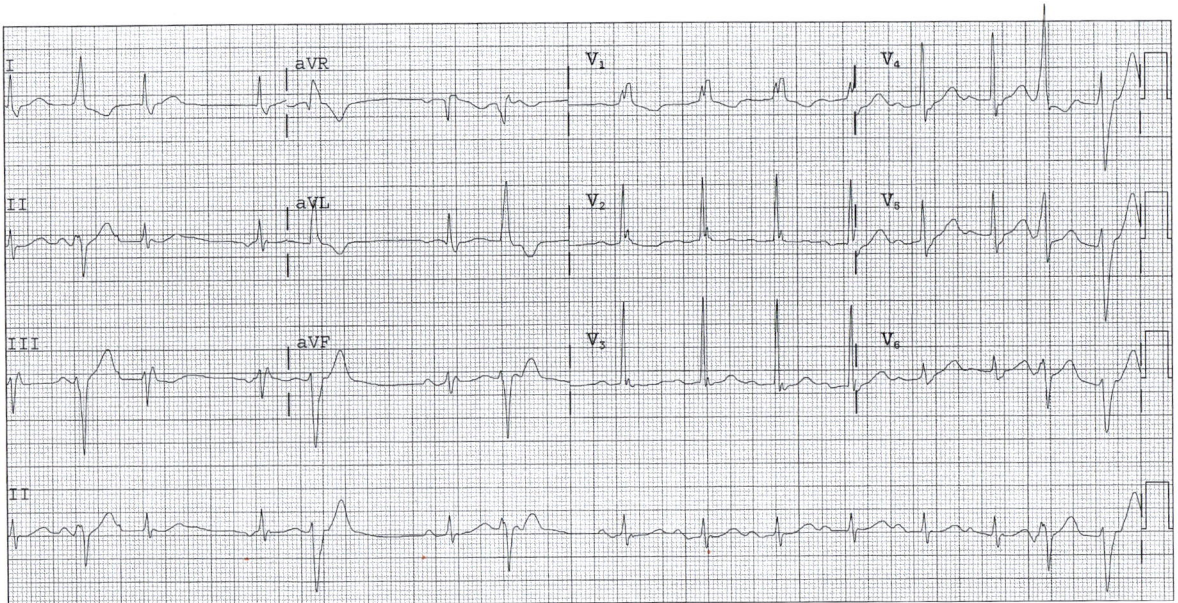

Figure 3.10a

CASE STUDY ON ECG 10

A patient with long-standing lung disease presents with worsening dyspnoea. Upon further assessment an ECG was obtained.

Please interpret the ECG in Figure 3.10a in a systematic manner.

Rhythm _____

Rate _____

Axis _____

P wave _____

PR interval _____

QRS complex _____

ST segment _____

T wave morphology _____

QT interval _____

Conclusion _____

Clinical notes _____

Diagnosis _____

_____

_____

_____

_____

Further investigations _____

_____

_____

_____

Management _____

_____

_____

_____

_____

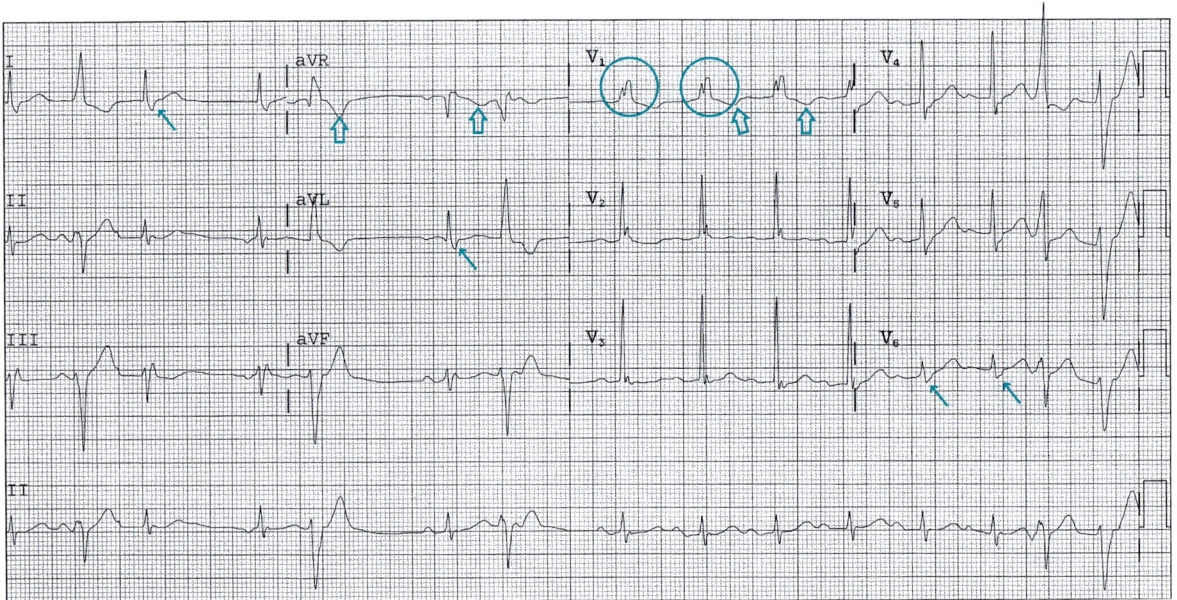

Figure 3.10b Right bundle branch block

ANSWER TO CASE STUDY ON ECG 10: RIGHT BUNDLE BRANCH BLOCK

A

The patient is in sinus rhythm. The rate is 96 bpm. The axis remains normal at −4° (Fig 3.10b).

The QRS complex is widened at a duration of 140 ms.

The features in the precordial leads are consistent with RBBB, including:

- rSR pattern in lead V_1 with prominent second R wave after the S wave (circles)
- Terminal S waves in leads I, aVL and V_6 (thin arrows)
- Note that in classic RBBB, the first r wave in the QRS complex of V_1 appears more prominent (R′SR). Thus it is also reasonable to call the RBBB in this ECG 'partial'

- T wave inversion and ST segment depression can be seen in V_1 and aVR (thick arrows)
- ST segment elevation can sometimes be seen in leads V_5 and/or V_6: discordant ST segment shift.

RBBB pattern can be seen in chronic lung disease.

RBBB can also present without any cardiac pathology as a normal variant (in contrast, LBBB pattern is always due to an underlying pathology).

Another feature to note in this ECG are the VEBs that are of two different morphologies indicating that they originate from different foci within the ventricles.

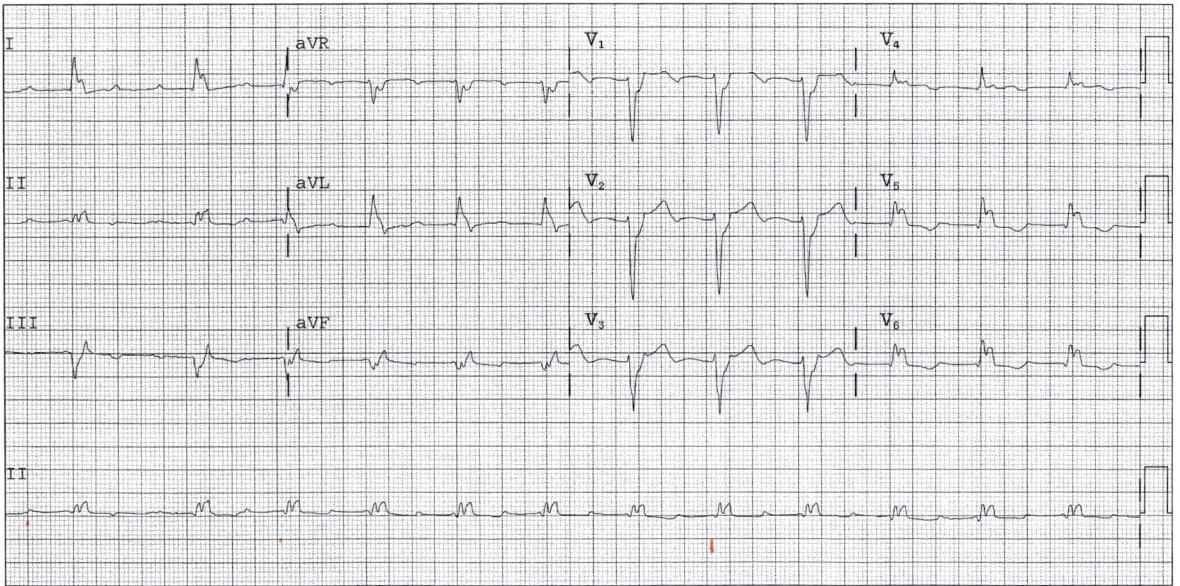

Figure 3.11a

CASE STUDY ON ECG 11

An 80-year-old man presents with decreasing mobility. Upon further assessment an ECG was obtained.

Please interpret the ECG in Figure 3.11a in a systematic manner.

Rhythm _____

Rate _____

Axis _____

P wave _____

PR interval _____

QRS complex _____

ST segment _____

T wave morphology _____

QT interval _____

Conclusion _____

Clinical notes _____

Diagnosis _____

_____

_____

_____

Further investigations _____

_____

_____

_____

Management _____

_____

_____

_____

_____

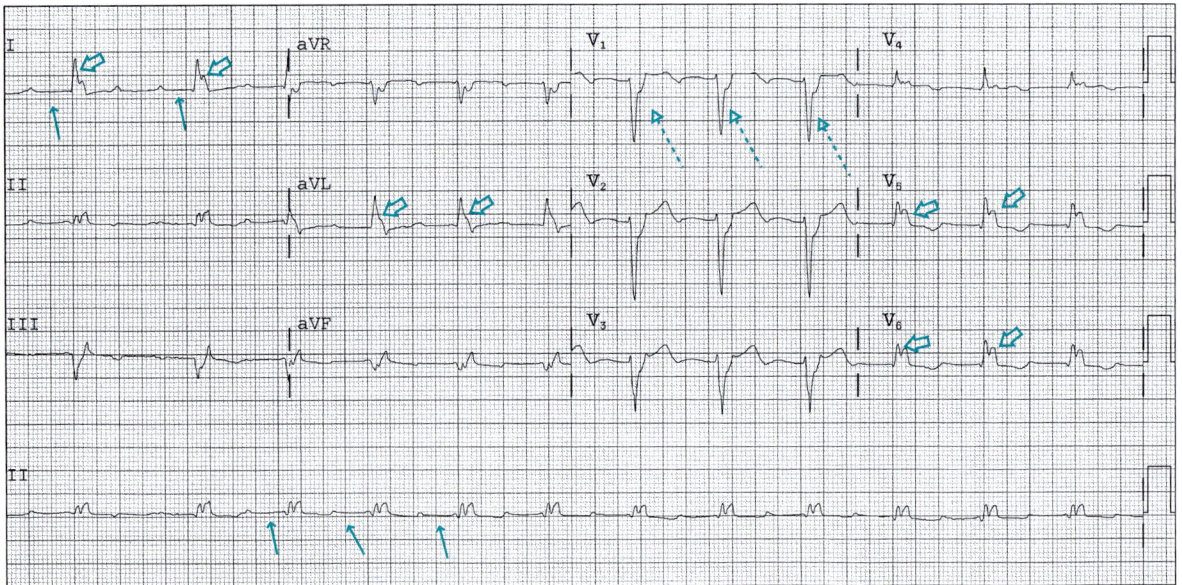

Figure 3.11b First degree heart block in trifascicular block

ANSWER TO CASE STUDY ON ECG 11: FIRST DEGREE HEART BLOCK IN TRIFASCICULAR BLOCK

A

Note the rhythm is regular and sinus. The rate is 76 bpm (Fig 3.11b). The axis is normal at $-5°$. There is prolongation of the PR interval (373 ms) (thin arrows) indicating first degree heart block.

The QRS complex duration is 173 ms. The QRS complex is wide and the morphology of the QRS complexes in the precordial or chest leads suggests a left bundle branch block (LBBB). Note the features of LBBB: wide QRS complex with a duration of more than 120 ms.

There are prominent and wide R waves in leads I, V_5, V_6 and aVL (thick arrows).

Note the prominent S wave or QS complex in lead V_1 (broken arrows).

There is poor R wave progression in leads V_1 to V_3.

There is also ST segment depression in the leads V_5 and V_6 with T wave inversion consistent with discordant ST segment shift.

Also note ST segment elevation in leads V_2 and V_3 that is concave upwards. This is an associated feature of LBBB.

Remember that the left bundle has two fascicles. In this ECG there are conduction blocks in the pathway between the sinoatrial node and the AV node (first degree heart block) and in the two fascicles of the left bundle (LBBB), hence it is called trifascicular block. This situation is equivalent to complete heart block. This patient may benefit from a permanent pacemaker implantation.

The aetiology of cardiac conduction defects in the elderly is degenerative unless there are clear features of coronary ischaemia.

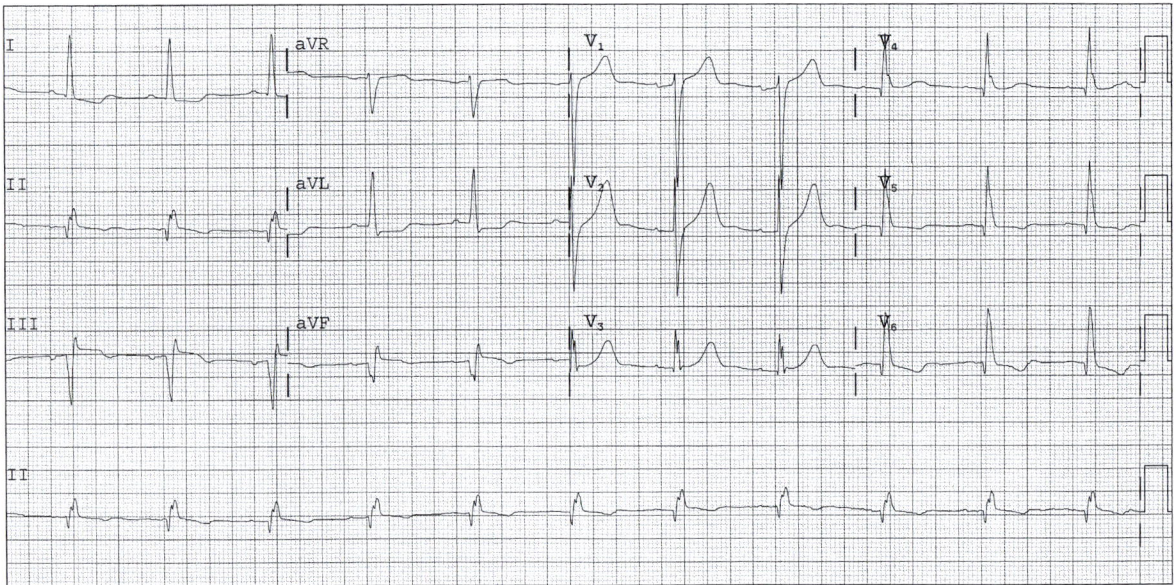

Figure 3.12a

CASE STUDY ON ECG 12

An 82-year-old woman presents with epigastric pain, nausea and vomiting. She was diaphoretic and hypotensive on presentation. She has a history of hypertension. Upon further assessment an ECG was obtained.

Please interpret the ECG in Figure 3.12a in a systematic manner.

Rhythm _____

Rate _____

Axis _____

P wave _____

PR interval _____

QRS complex _____

ST segment _____

T wave morphology _____

QT interval _____

Conclusion _____

Clinical notes _____

Diagnosis _____

_____

_____

_____

_____

Further investigations _____

_____

_____

_____

Management _____

_____

_____

_____

_____

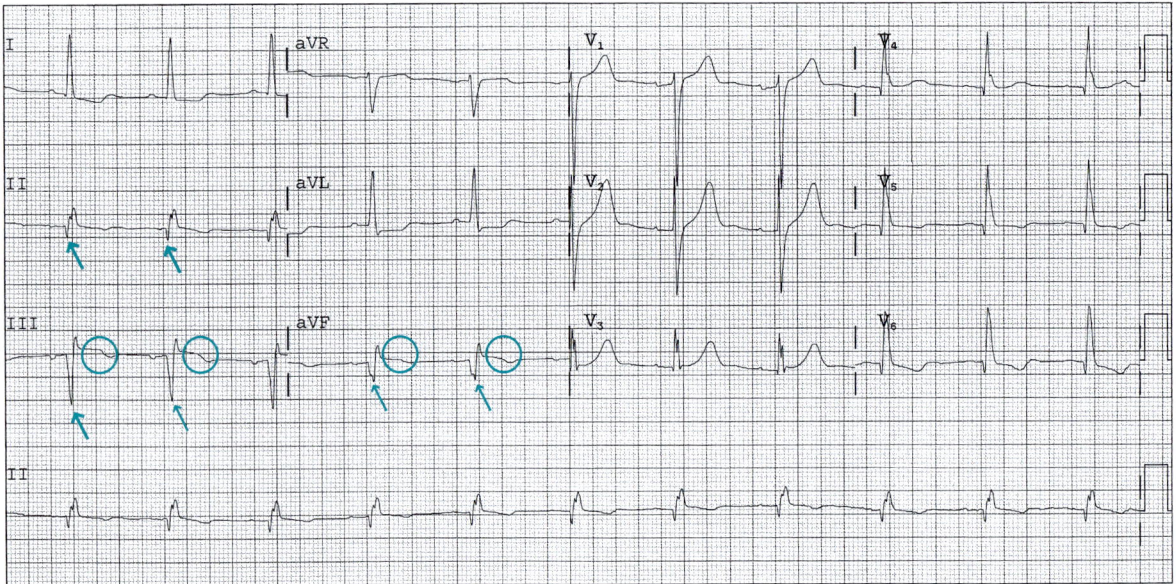

Figure 3.12b Inferior STEMI

ANSWER TO CASE STUDY ON ECG 12: INFERIOR STEMI

A

Heart rate is 70 bpm. The rhythm is regular. The axis is normal (Fig 3.12b).

The striking abnormality is the ST segment elevation seen in leads III and aVF (circles), together with T wave inversion in the inferior and lateral leads. These features together with the presenting clinical picture are consistent with an acute ST segment elevation myocardial infarction (STEMI). Occlusion of the right coronary artery causes 90 per cent of inferior infarcts. Inferior infarcts usually present with associated nausea and vomiting. Note that female patients may present with atypical chest pain in the setting of myocardial infarction as

this woman did. Note the formation of Q waves in the inferior leads (arrows). The formation of Q waves indicates that the infarction has evolved, possibly due to late presentation after the onset of chest pain.

The patient also shows evidence of left ventricular hypertrophy (LVH): tall R waves in aVL, deep S waves in leads V_1 and V_2 together with tall R waves in leads V_5 and V_6. T wave inversion in leads I, V_5 and V_6 could be due to LVH and/or ischaemia.

This patient needs urgent stabilisation and referral for primary angioplasty or thrombolysis to reopen the completely occluded artery.

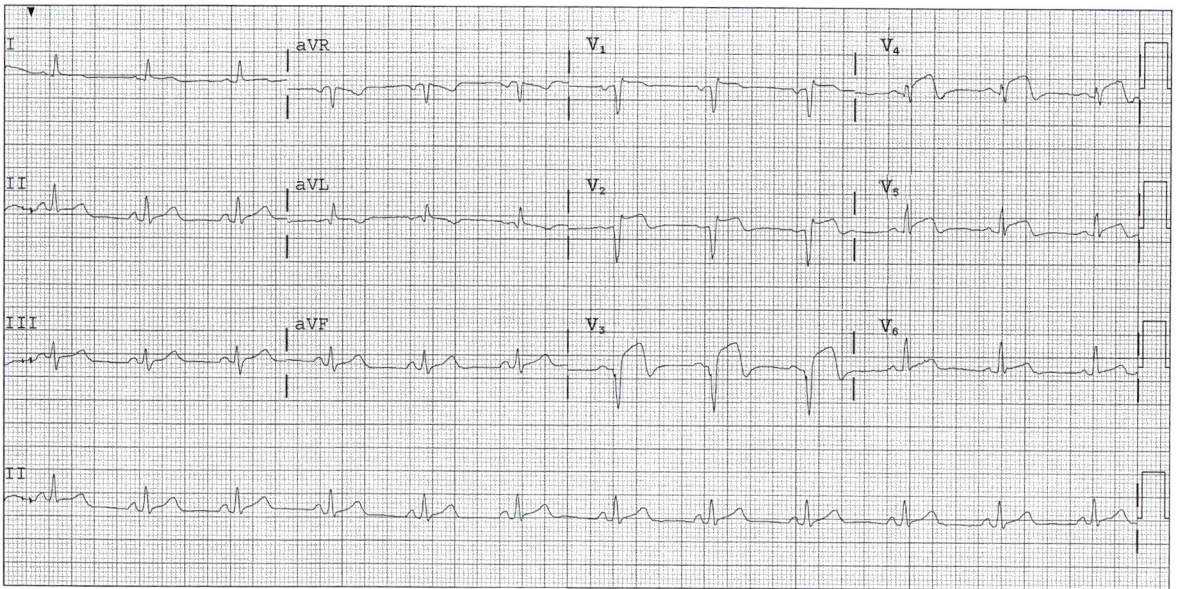

Figure 3.13a

CASE STUDY ON ECG 13

A 53-year-old smoker presents with severe retrosternal chest tightness and diaphoresis. On examination he has a mid-diastolic murmur. Upon further assessment an ECG was obtained.

Please interpret the ECG in Figure 3.13a in a systematic manner.

Rhythm _____

Rate _____

Axis _____

P wave _____

PR interval _____

QRS complex _____

ST segment _____

T wave morphology _____

QT interval _____

Conclusion _____

Clinical notes _____

Diagnosis _____

_____

_____

_____

_____

Further investigations _____

_____

_____

_____

_____

Management _____

_____

_____

_____

_____

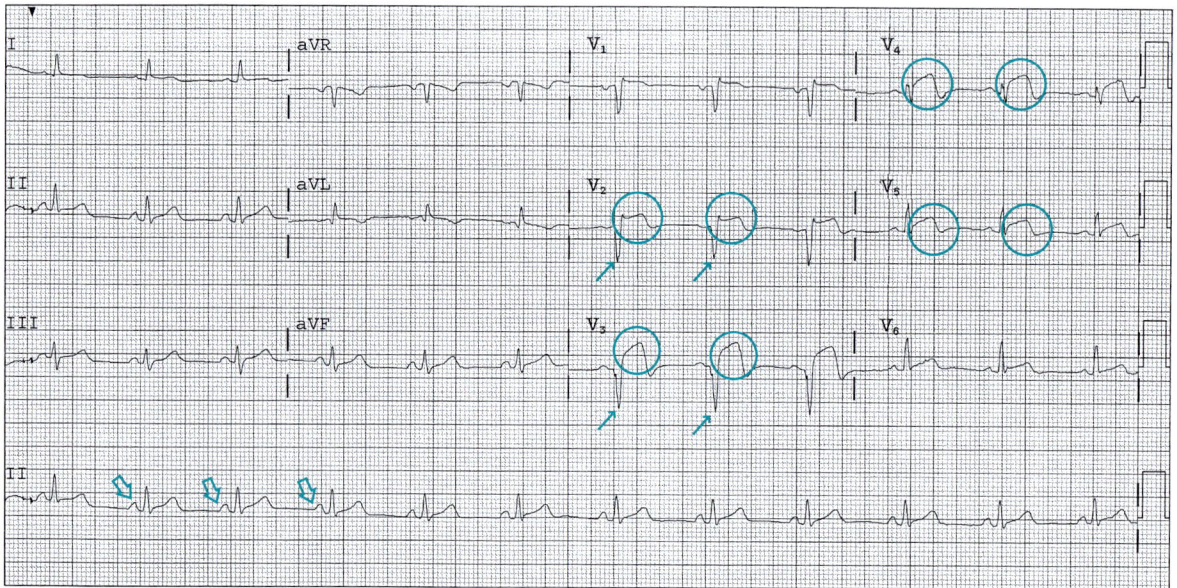

Figure 3.13b STEMI with background LA enlargement

ANSWER TO CASE STUDY ON ECG 13: STEMI WITH BACKGROUND ANTEROLATERAL ENLARGEMENT

Note the rate is 75 bpm and the rhythm is regular. The axis is normal (Fig 3.13b).

The striking abnormality is the ST segment elevation seen in the leads V_2, V_3, V_4 and V_5, indicating an anterolateral STEMI. There are Q waves formed in leads V_2 and V_3 (thin arrows).

This patient needs urgent stabilisation and referral for urgent primary angioplasty to reopen the occluded left anterior descending (LAD) artery.

Also note the prominent P waves in lead II and several other leads (thick arrows). The duration of the P wave in lead II is close to 120 ms (3 small squares). This may suggest left atrial hypertrophy. This is in keeping with the fact that the patient has a mid-diastolic murmur probably due to mitral valve stenosis, a condition that can cause left atrial hypertrophy. To investigate this, the patient needs further assessment with echocardiography.

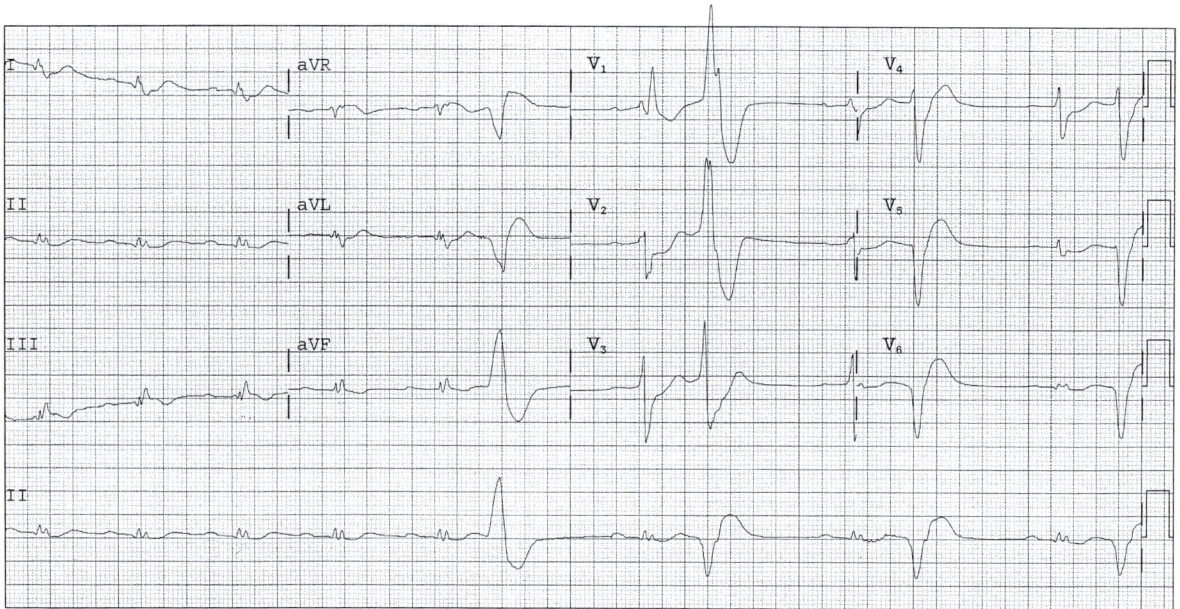

Figure 3.14a

CASE STUDY ON ECG 14

Q

A 76-year-old man presents with chest tightness of half-hour duration. He is a smoker. Upon further assessment an ECG was obtained.

Please interpret the ECG in Figure 3.14a in a systematic manner.

Rhythm _____

Rate _____

Axis _____

P wave _____

PR interval _____

QRS complex _____

ST segment _____

T wave morphology _____

QT interval _____

Conclusion _____

Clinical notes _____

Diagnosis _____

_____

_____

_____

_____

Further investigations _____

_____

_____

_____

_____

Management _____

_____

_____

_____

_____

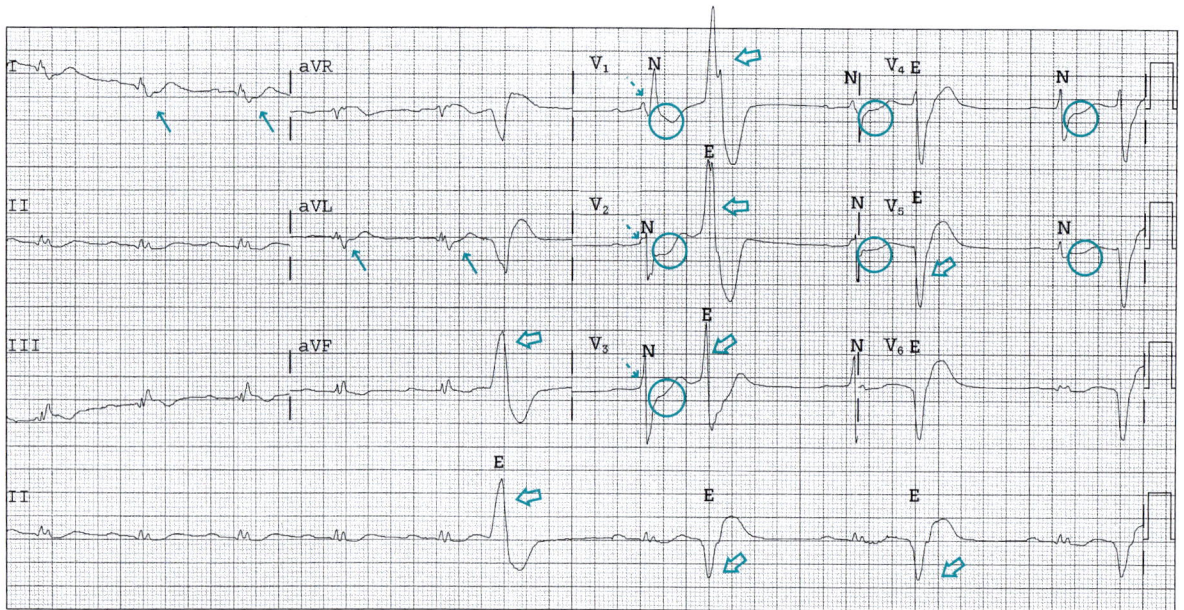

Figure 3.14b Posterior STEMI

ANSWER TO CASE STUDY ON ECG 14: POSTERIOR STEMI

The rate is 60 bpm and the rhythm is regular (Fig 3.14b). The axis is within normal limits.

This interesting ECG shows multiple abnormalities. Most important is the significant ST segment depression seen in leads V_1, V_2, V_3, V_4 and V_5 (circles), after the native (marked as N) QRS complexes. This is highly suggestive of a posterior wall myocardial infarction. The diagnosis should be suspected given the clinical information related to the presentation. There is mild ST segment depression in leads I and aVL (thin arrows), also in keeping with posterior wall infarct. There are tall R waves (dotted arrows) in the leads V_1, V_2 and V_3.

Do the mirror test by flipping the sheet over and turning it upside down (see Fig 1.31). Now look at it from the blank side of the paper against a bright light and notice the above changes of tall R waves appearing as Q waves, and the ST segment depression as ST segment elevations!

If you do a posterior ECG, you will see ST segment elevation in the leads V_7 to V_9.

This ECG shows ventricular ectopic beats of multiple different origins (thick arrows and marked as E). You should distinguish the native QRS complexes (marked as N) from these to further analyse the ST segments.

Native QRS complexes are broad and demonstrate RBBB pattern. Ventricular ectopic beats are of various different morphologies.

If the posterior ECG confirms the diagnosis, he needs to be stabilised with anticoagulants and antiplatelet agents and referred for urgent cardiac catheterisation. Where this facility is not available, thrombolysis is indicated, if safe.

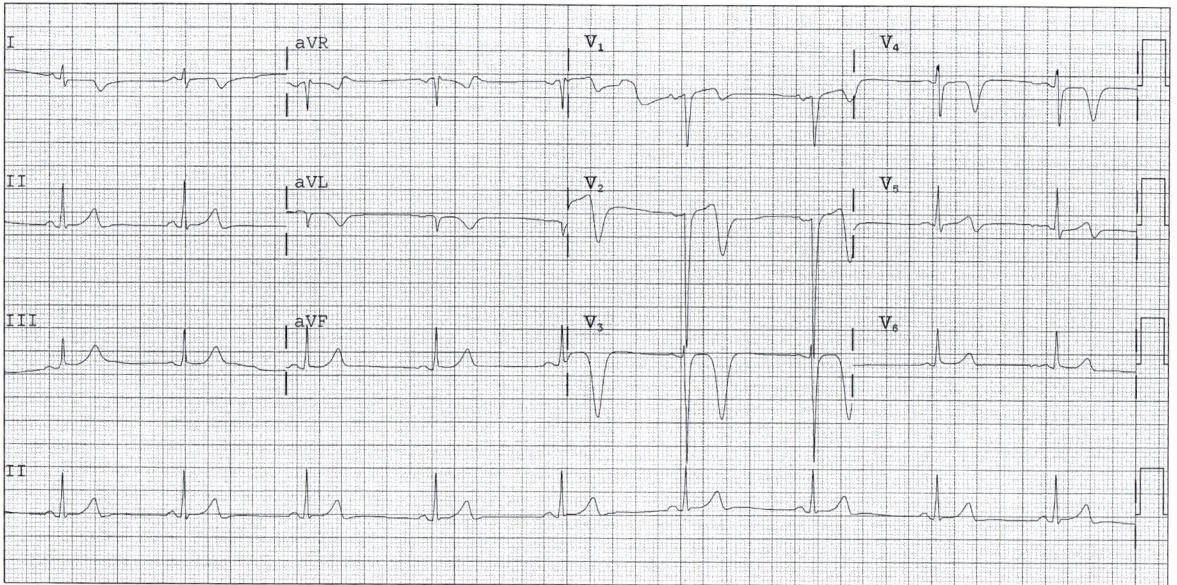

Figure 3.15a

CASE STUDY ON ECG 15

This 45-year-old man presents with chest pain at minimal exertion. He has had chest pain over a period of a few weeks, gradually increasing in severity and frequency. Upon further assessment an ECG was obtained. At the time of this ECG he had chest pain at rest. He has a strong family history of coronary artery disease.

Please interpret the ECG in Figure 3.15a in a systematic manner.

Rhythm _____

Rate _____

Axis _____

P wave _____

PR interval _____

QRS complex _____

ST segment _____

T wave morphology _____

QT interval _____

Conclusion _____

Clinical notes _____

Diagnosis _____

_____

_____

_____

_____

Further investigations _____

_____

_____

_____

_____

Management _____

_____

_____

_____

_____

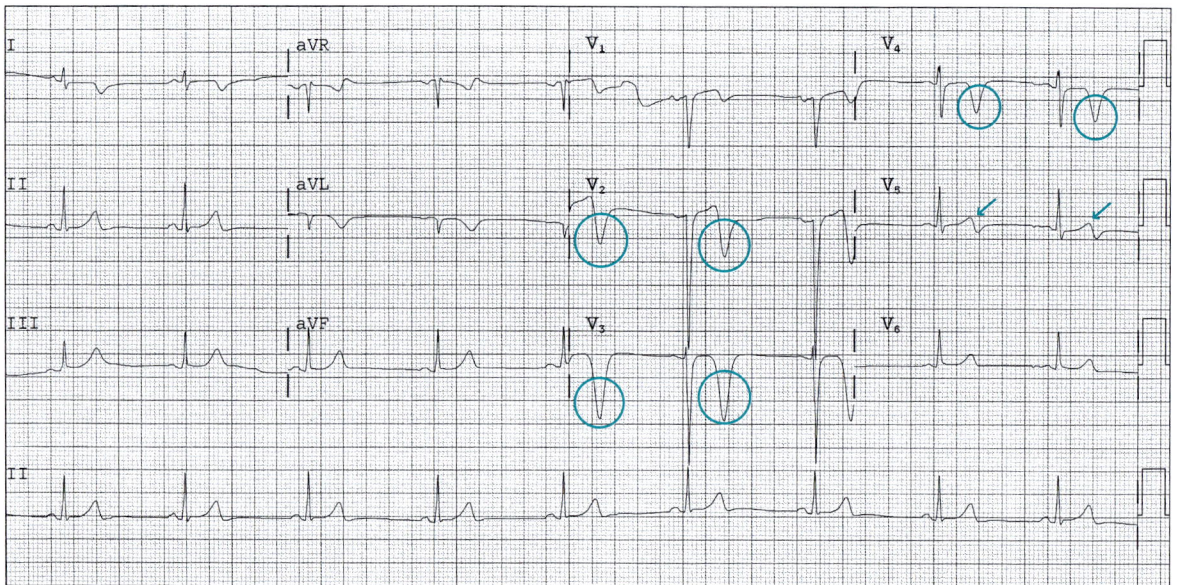

Figure 3.15b Wellens syndrome

ANSWER TO CASE STUDY ON ECG 15: WELLENS SYNDROME

A

The rhythm is regular and sinus. Heart rate is 55 bpm (Fig 3.15b). The axis is within normal limits.

The most striking feature is the deep T wave inversion seen in the leads V_2, V_3 and V_4 (circles). There is a biphasic T wave in the lead V_5 (thin arrows). There is mild ST segment elevation in leads V_1 and V_2.

Remember the salient features of Wellens syndrome:

- Deep T wave inversion in leads V_1 to V_4 and occasionally in V_5 and V_6 (sometimes deep T wave inversion could be limited to only V_2 and V_3) (the sloping angle of the inverted T wave is 60°–90° and it is symmetrical in morphology)
- Rarely instead of deep inversion, the T wave may appear biphasic in V_3 to V_5
- ST segments remain isoelectric or mildly elevated (around 1 mm).

This man is at very high risk of an ST segment elevation infarct (STEMI) of the anterior zone due to a high-grade occlusion of the left anterior descending (LAD) coronary artery. Hence he needs to be stabilised with anticoagulant therapy and antiplatelet therapy with referral for urgent or early cardiac catheterisation.

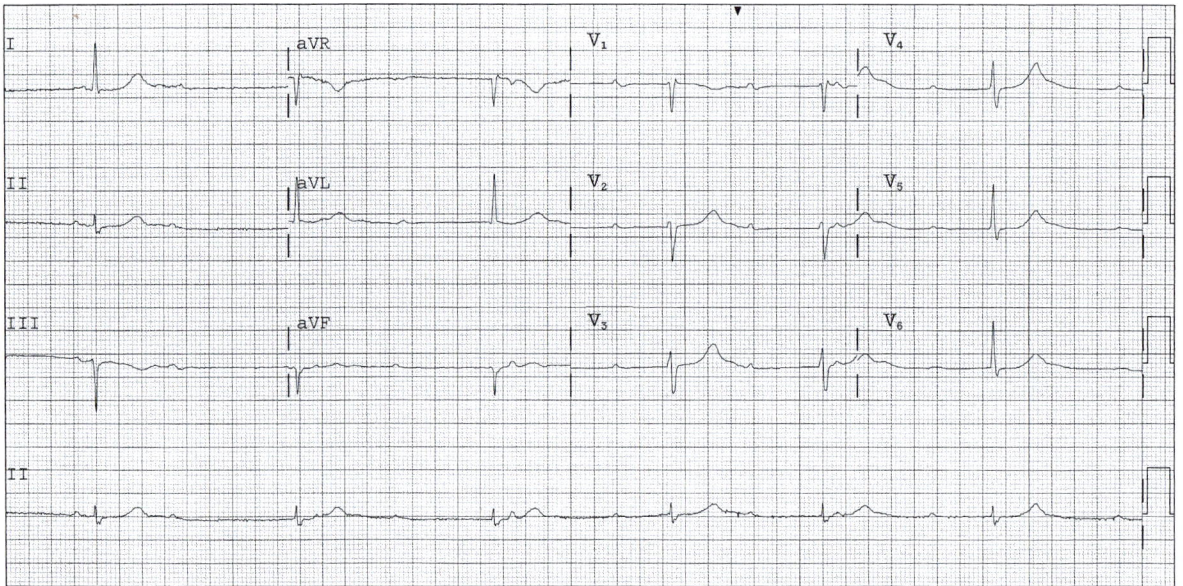

Figure 3.16a

CASE STUDY ON ECG 16

This 81-year-old woman had been experiencing chest tightness for a few days but failed to seek medical help. She was brought into the hospital after an episode of syncope. Her blood pressure was 70/40 mmHg. Upon further assessment an ECG was obtained.

Please interpret the ECG in Figure 3.16a in a systematic manner.

Rhythm _____

Rate _____

Axis _____

P wave _____

PR interval _____

QRS complex _____

ST segment _____

T wave morphology _____

QT interval _____

Conclusion _____

Clinical notes _____

Diagnosis _____

_____

_____

_____

Further investigations _____

_____

_____

_____

Management _____

_____

_____

_____

_____

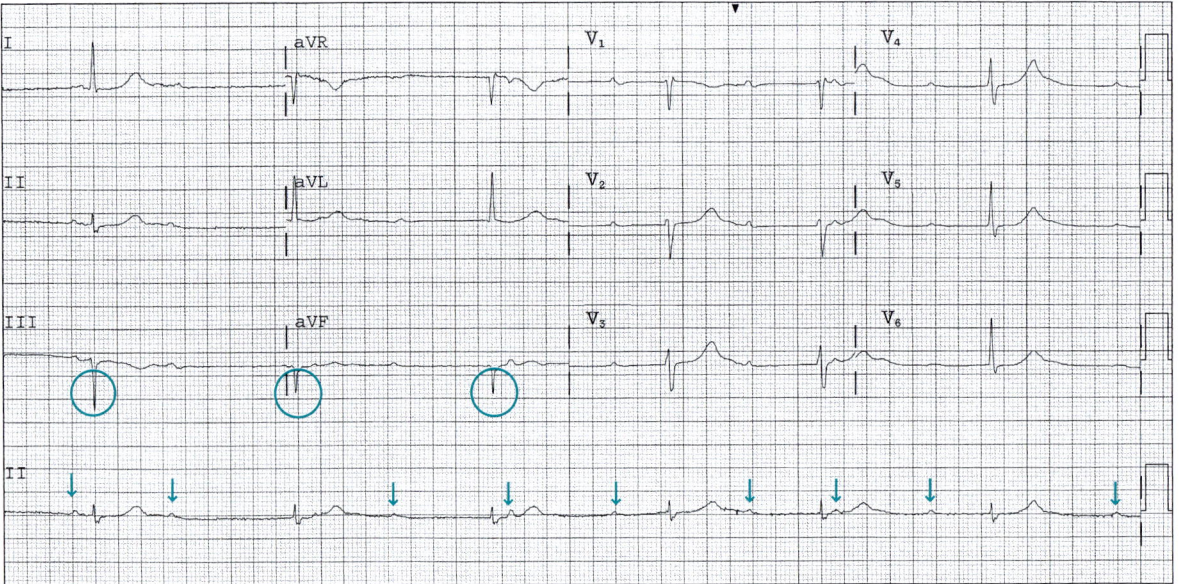

Figure 3.16b Bradycardia

ANSWER TO CASE STUDY ON ECG 16: BRADYCARDIA

A

Note that the rate is less than 40 bpm indicating severe bradycardia. The rhythm is irregular (Fig 3.16b). The axis is deviated to the left.

The P waves (arrows) have no clear relationship to the QRS complexes. QRS complexes are not wide. Also note that the P waves are not regular. This is complete heart block with a junctional escape rhythm. The fact that the QRS complex is narrow indicates that the escape rhythm is originating above the level of the ventricle. If it were of ventricular origin the QRS complex would be wider than 120 ms.

Also note the Q waves in the inferior region (circles) in the leads III and aVF. This indicates previous inferior infarction.

This patient may have had her infarction in the preceding days when she experienced the chest pain. She has subsequently developed complete heart block due to occlusion of the artery that supplies the AV node, which is the posterior descending coronary artery (PDA). In 90 per cent of the population this artery is a branch of the right coronary artery.

This patient needs haemodynamic stability established with the insertion of a temporary pacemaker. Another way to accelerate the slow heart rate is to administer an infusion of isoprenaline. In the presence of coronary ischaemia, this should be done with extreme caution. Isoprenaline infusion can exacerbate coronary ischaemia. She may benefit from coronary angiography to reopen the occluded PDA. Upon reopening of the coronary artery, if her heart block is not resolved she may require a permanent pacemaker implantation.

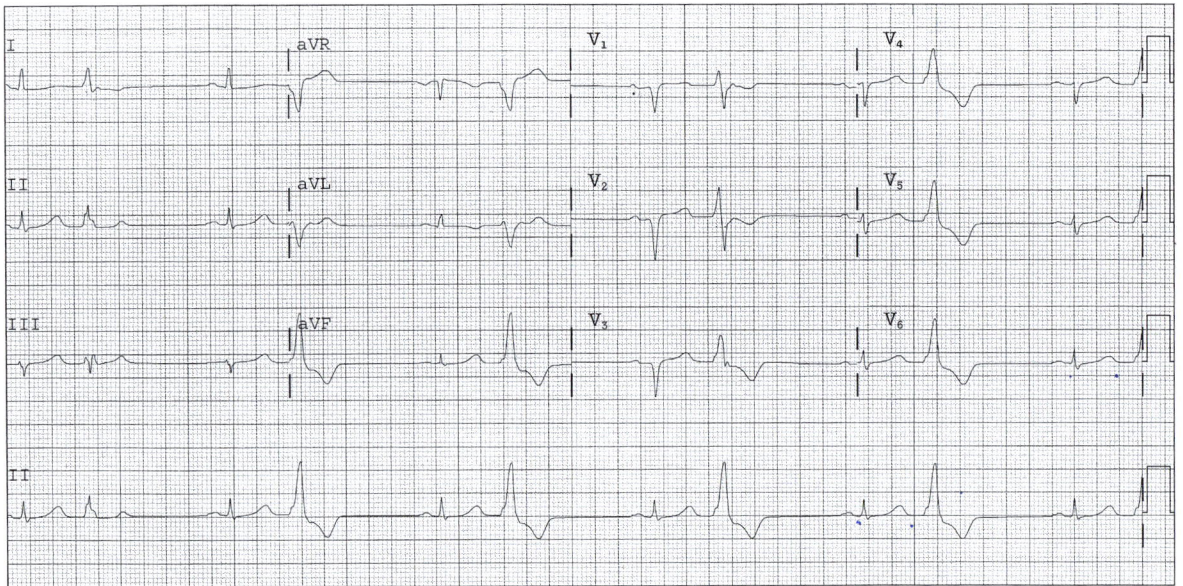

Figure 3.17a

CASE STUDY ON ECG 17

This 50-year-old woman presents with dyspnoea and palpitations. She has a past history of coronary artery disease. Upon further assessment an ECG was obtained.

Please interpret the ECG in Figure 3.17a in a systematic manner.

Rhythm _____

Rate _____

Axis _____

P wave _____

PR interval _____

QRS complex _____

ST segment _____

T wave morphology _____

QT interval _____

Conclusion _____

Clinical notes _____

Diagnosis _____

_____

_____

_____

Further investigations _____

_____

_____

_____

Management _____

_____

_____

_____

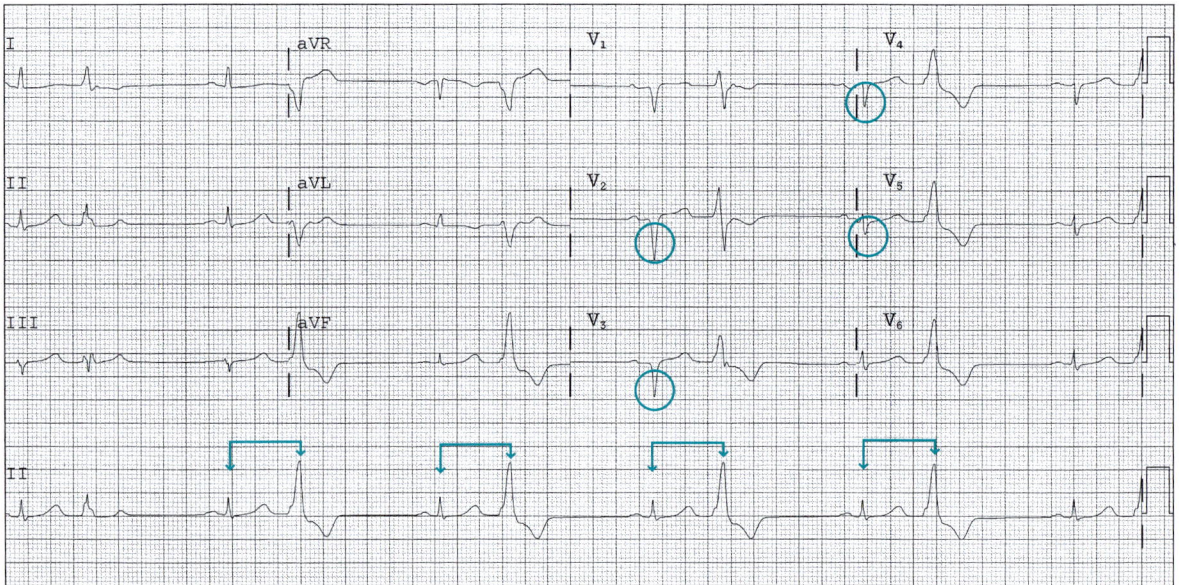

Figure 3.17b Ventricular bigeminy

ANSWER TO CASE STUDY ON ECG 17: VENTRICULAR BIGEMINY

A

Note that the rate is 74 bpm. The rhythm is regularly irregular. The axis is normal (Fig 3.17b).

Note that each narrow QRS complex is followed immediately by a broad QRS complex (paired arrows). The narrow complex is preceded by a P wave, hence it is a sinus complex. The wide complex is a ventricular complex. This phenomenon of regular sinus complex paired with a ventricular complex is called (atrio) ventricular bigeminy.

Also note the Q waves in the septal and lateral leads (V_2 to V_5) (circles). This may indicate a previous myocardial infarction. Remember, this patient has a history of coronary artery disease.

The native (sinus) QRS complexes are not followed by T wave inversion or ST segment depression. Hence there is no evidence of acute coronary ischaemia despite her past history to this effect.

The AV bigeminy may have contributed to her feeling of palpitation. If she maintains a good blood pressure this abnormality does not require any specific treatment currently.

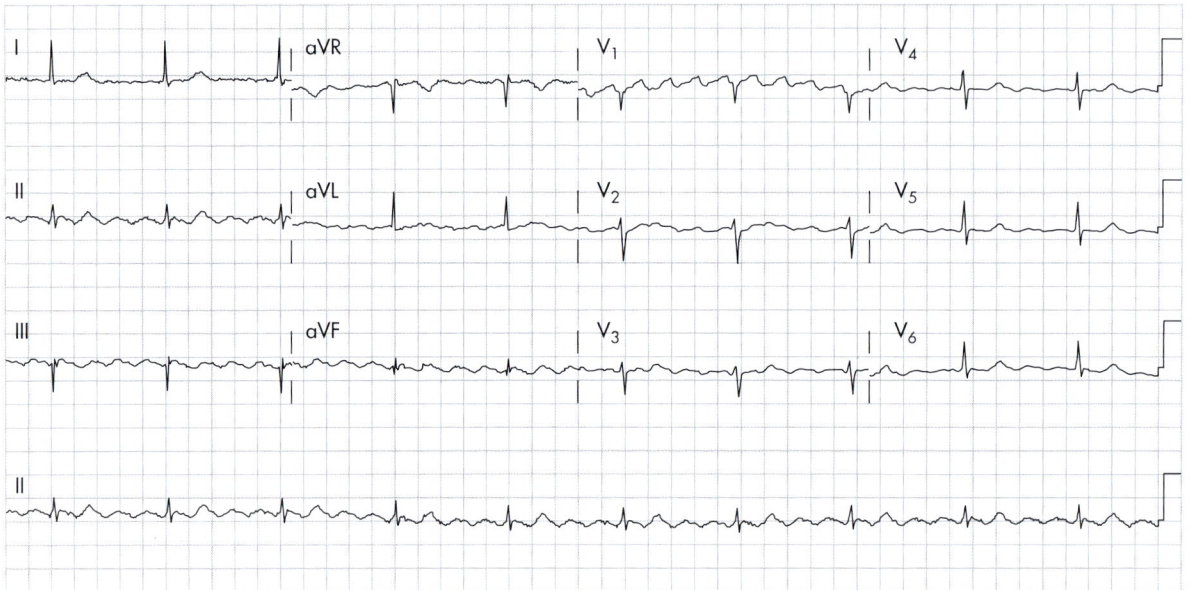

Figure 3.18a

CASE STUDY ON ECG 18

This 49-year-old woman presents with palpitations and 'light headedness'. She has had an alcohol binge the previous night. Upon further assessment an ECG was obtained.

Please interpret the ECG in Figure 3.18a in a systematic manner.

Rhythm _____

Rate _____

Axis _____

P wave _____

PR interval _____

QRS complex _____

ST segment _____

T wave morphology _____

QT interval _____

Conclusion _____

Clinical notes _____

Diagnosis _____

_____

_____

_____

_____

Further investigations _____

_____

_____

_____

_____

Management _____

_____

_____

_____

_____

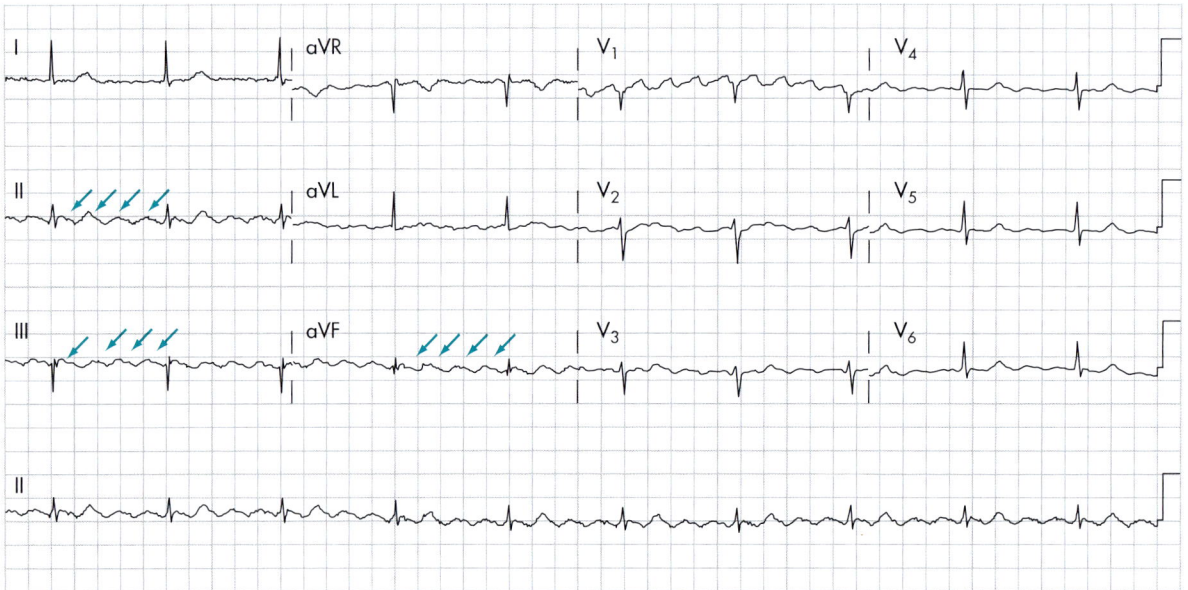

Figure 3.18b Atrial flutter

ANSWER TO CASE STUDY ON ECG 18: ATRIAL FLUTTER

A

Note that the rate is around 61 bpm. The rhythm is regular. The axis is normal (Fig 3.18b).

Note the saw-tooth shaped P (flutter) waves best seen in leads II, III and aVF (arrows) and less conspicuously in the other leads. The rate of these flutter waves is 300 per minute; this is a classic feature of atrial flutter.

The ventricular response is at a slower rate than that of the atria. Out of every four atrial beats only one is conducted to the ventricle, hence this is called atrial flutter with a 4 : 1 AV block. Usually when there is atrial flutter with 4 : 1 block the rate is 75 bpm, but in this case it is 61 bpm.

Ventricular response to atrial flutter can vary depending on the degree of AV block. When the block is 2 : 1 the ventricular rate will be 150 bpm, and when it is 3 : 1 it will be 100 bpm. The rapid heart rate may have caused the patient's blood pressure to drop leading to the feeling of presyncope. However the rate has settled to a satisfactory level now.

The patient needs medications to maintain rate control as well as to achieve rhythm control. Atrial flutter can evolve to atrial fibrillation. Assess the patient's risk of thromboembolic stroke by taking into consideration other risk factors, such as hypertension, congestive cardiac failure, diabetes mellitus or previous stroke if present.

If the patient is significantly unstable due to flutter or fibrillation, urgent (DC) electrical cardioversion is required. Atrial flutter can also be treated with radiofrequency ablation.

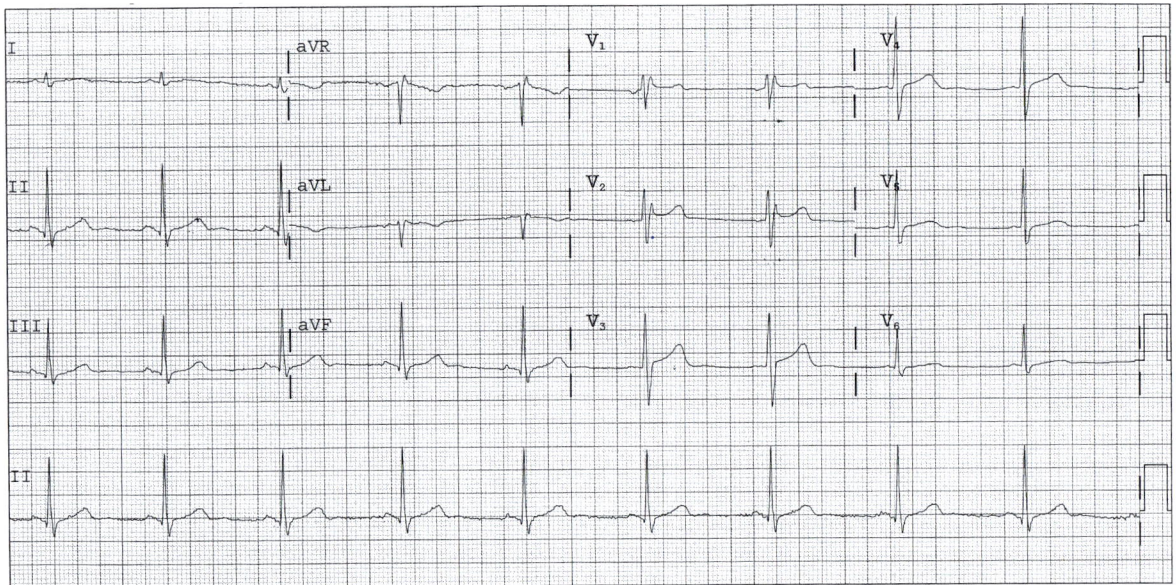

Figure 3.19a

CASE STUDY ON ECG 19

This 59-year-old man presents with general malaise. He is a smoker with a history of diabetes. Upon further assessment an ECG was obtained.

Please interpret the ECG in Figure 3.19a in a systematic manner.

Rhythm _____

Rate _____

Axis _____

P wave _____

PR interval _____

QRS complex _____

ST segment _____

T wave morphology _____

QT interval _____

Conclusion _____

Clinical notes _____

Diagnosis _____

_____

_____

_____

_____

Further investigations _____

_____

_____

_____

Management _____

_____

_____

_____

_____

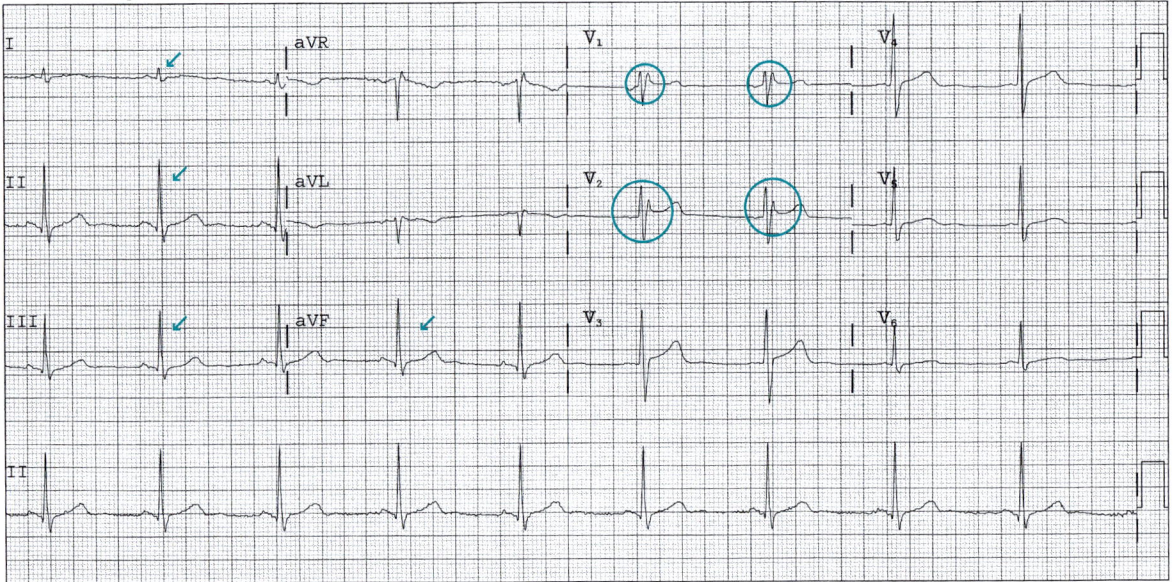

Figure 3.19b Right bundle branch block

ANSWER TO CASE STUDY ON ECG 19: RIGHT BUNDLE BRANCH BLOCK

A

Note that the rate is 56 bpm. The rhythm is regular (Fig 3.19b).

The axis is normal but more towards the +90° direction (closer to the right side but not quite). QRS complex is predominantly upwards in leads II, III and aVF (arrows). It remains upwards also in lead I (arrow).

Note the RSR morphology of the QRS complex in leads V_1 and V_2 that is also wide in duration (circles). However the QRS complex remains normal in the other leads. This is

suggestive of a partial or incomplete right bundle branch block (RBBB).

There is minor ST segment elevation in leads V_1, V_2 and V_3 but not quite severe enough to indicate coronary ischaemia. Usually coronary ischaemia is confirmed when the ST segment elevation in the anterior precordial leads is more than 2 mm.

This patient needs to be further observed to ensure that there is no further progression of ECG changes.

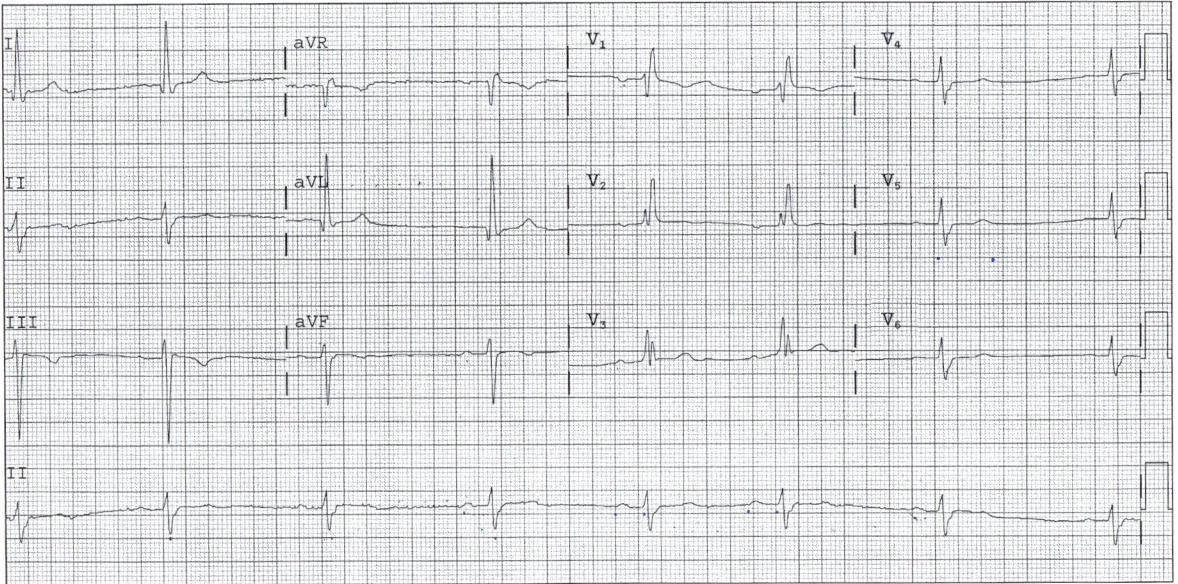

Figure 3.20a

CASE STUDY ON ECG 20

An 80-year-old man presents with fatigue and light headedness. He is not taking any medication that would cause bradycardia. Upon further assessment an ECG was obtained.

Please interpret the ECG in Figure 3.20a in a systematic manner.

Rhythm _____

Rate _____

Axis _____

P wave _____

PR interval _____

QRS complex _____

ST segment _____

T wave morphology _____

QT interval _____

Conclusion _____

Clinical notes _____

Diagnosis _____

_____

_____

_____

_____

Further investigations _____

_____

_____

_____

Management _____

_____

_____

_____

_____

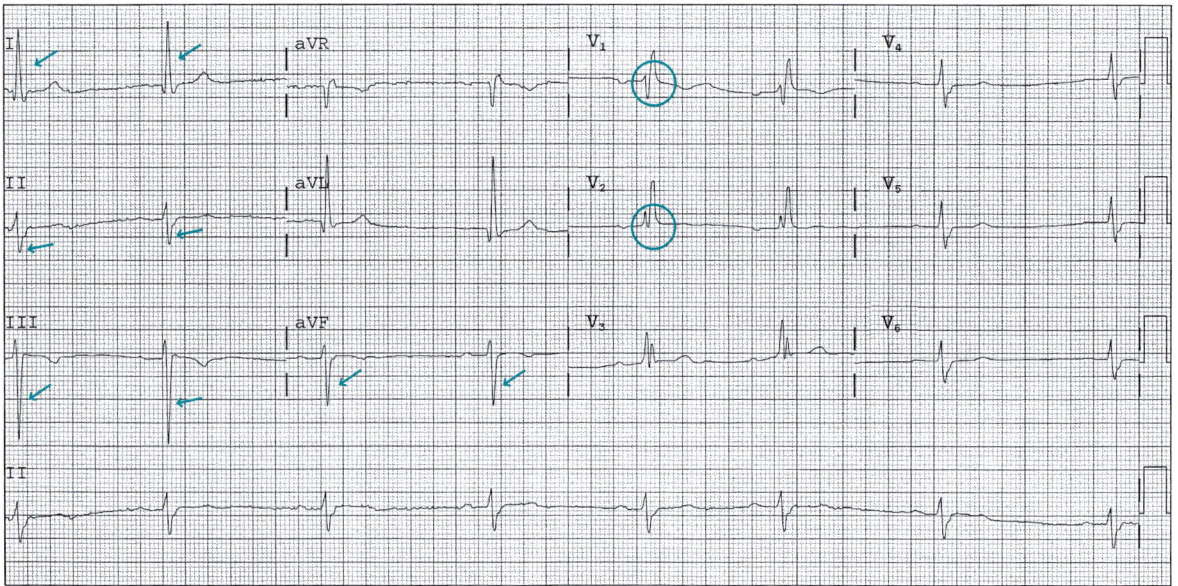

Figure 3.20b Trifascicular block

ANSWER TO CASE STUDY ON ECG 20: TRIFASCICULAR BLOCK

A

Note the rhythm is regular but the rate is 45 bpm indicating bradycardia (Fig 3.20b).

The axis is to the left (left axis deviation (LAD)). The QRS complex is predominantly directed downwards in leads II, III and aVF (arrows). It is upwards in lead I (arrows). According to the two-leads method and the three-leads method you can estimate the axis to be to the left.

PR interval is longer than 200 ms, indicating first degree heart block. Also note the features of right bundle branch block. QRS complex is wider than 120 ms.

The features of RBBB include:

- The rSR pattern in leads V_1 and V_2 with prominent second R wave after the S wave (circles)
- Terminal S waves in leads I, aVL and V_6

- Note the qRS (with prominent S wave) complex in lead V_6
- There is a terminal R wave also in lead aVR.

T wave inversion and ST segment depression can be seen in V_1 and aVR.

LAD is indicative of left anterior fascicular block (LAFB). Note the axis is deviated to the left between $-90°$ and $-45°$.

Small q waves are seen in leads I and/or aVL; small r waves in inferior leads (II, III and aVF) together with prominent S waves (rS complexes in inferior leads). There are deep S waves in leads V_5 and V_6.

This patient with significant cardiac conduction defects and symptomatic bradycardia needs treatment with a permanent pacemaker implantation.

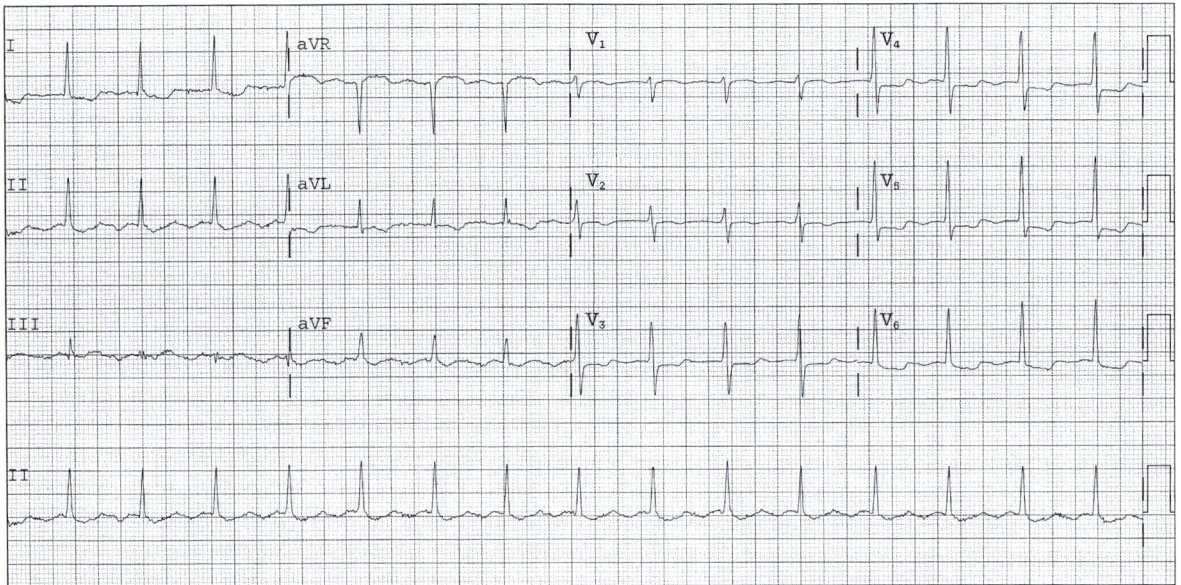

Figure 3.21a

CASE STUDY ON ECG 21

A 56-year-old man presents with chest pain at rest. Upon further assessment an ECG was obtained.

Please interpret the ECG in Figure 3.21a in a systematic manner.

Rhythm _____

Rate _____

Axis _____

P wave _____

PR interval _____

QRS complex _____

ST segment _____

T wave morphology _____

QT interval _____

Conclusion _____

Clinical notes _____

Diagnosis _____

_____

_____

_____

_____

Further investigations _____

_____

_____

_____

_____

Management _____

_____

_____

_____

_____

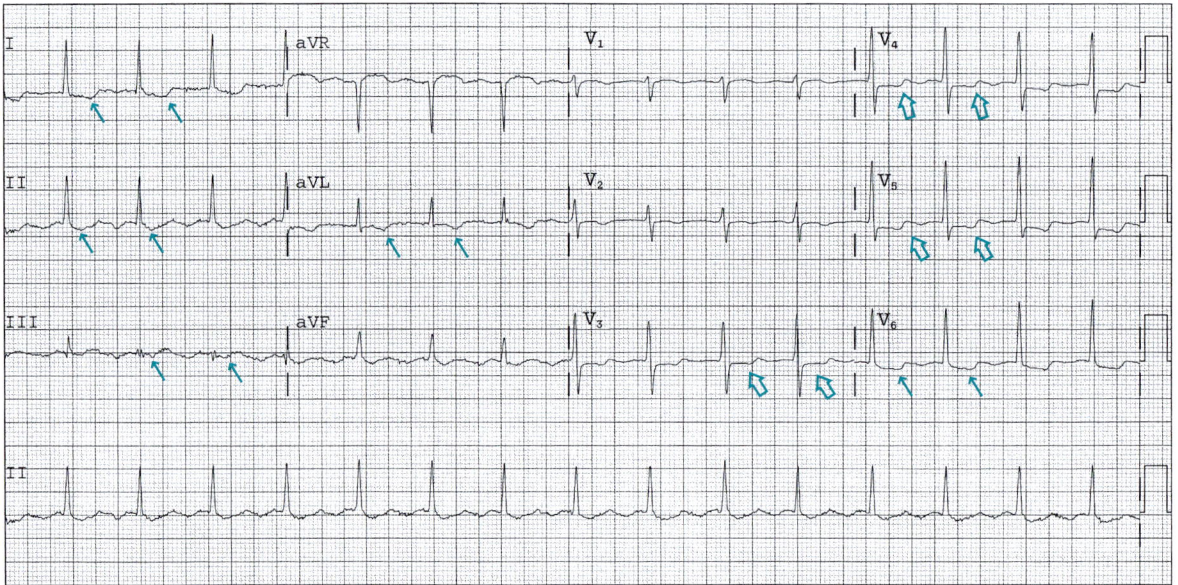

Figure 3.21b Accelerated junctional rhythm

ANSWER TO CASE STUDY ON ECG 21: ACCELERATED JUNCTIONAL RHYTHM

The rate is approximately 90 bpm. The rhythm is regular and the QRS complexes are not preceded by a P wave (P waves are absent). The axis is normal (Fig 3.21b).

The QRS complexes are narrow, hence not of ventricular origin. In the absence of P waves it is clear that the AV junctional node has taken over the pacemaker role. Usually the junctional escape rhythm has a much slower rate. But on this ECG the rate is faster so it is called an 'accelerated junctional escape rhythm'.

Note also the T wave inversions seen in leads I, II, III, aVL and V_6 (thin arrows).

There are biphasic T waves in the leads V_3, V_4 and V_5 (thick arrows).

In the presence of coronary risk factors and typical chest pain these changes are highly suggestive of diffuse and widespread coronary ischaemia.

This patient has acute coronary syndrome unless proven otherwise. He should be managed with anticoagulation therapy, antiplatelet therapy and nitrates for chest pain. He may benefit from early coronary angiography.

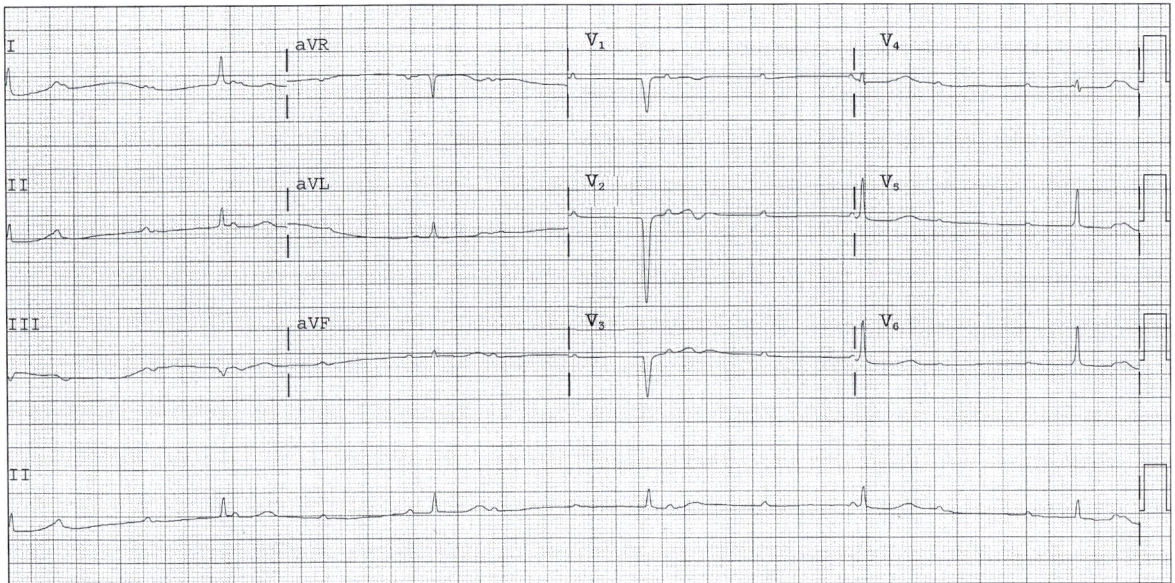

Figure 3.22a

CASE STUDY ON ECG 22

A 93-year-old man was brought in after collapsing at home. Upon further assessment this ECG was obtained.

Please interpret the ECG in Figure 3.22a in a systematic manner.

Rhythm _____

Rate _____

Axis _____

P wave _____

PR interval _____

QRS complex _____

ST segment _____

T wave morphology _____

QT interval _____

Conclusion _____

Clinical notes _____

Diagnosis _____

_____

_____

_____

_____

Further investigations _____

_____

_____

_____

_____

Management _____

_____

_____

_____

_____

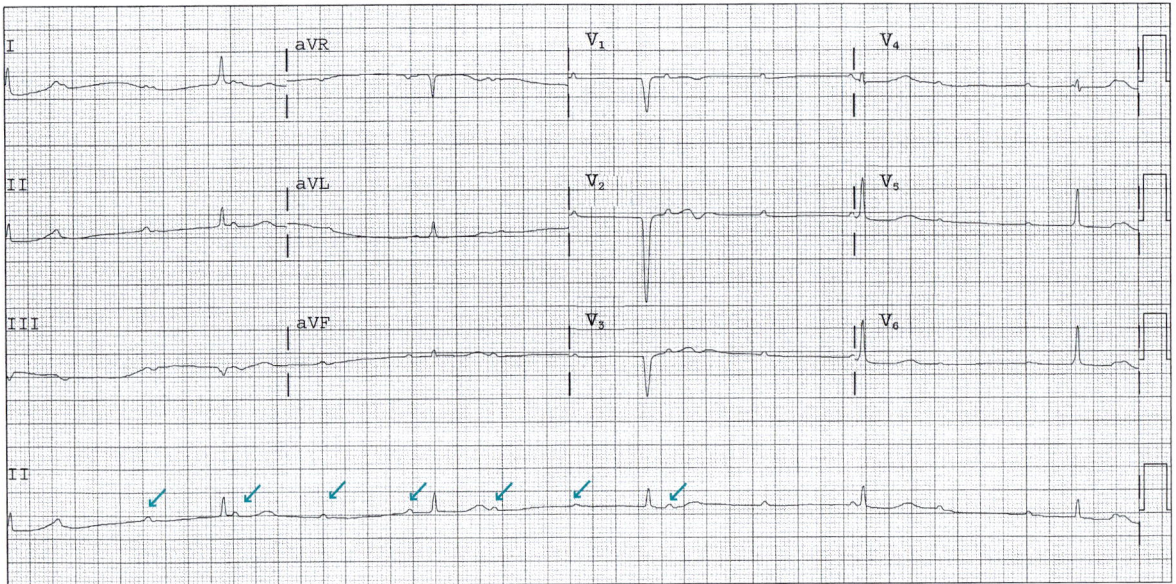

Figure 3.22b Complete heart block

ANSWER TO CASE STUDY ON ECG 22: COMPLETE HEART BLOCK

Note that the rate is approximately 30 bpm indicating severe bradycardia. The rhythm is regular. The axis is normal (Fig 3.22b).

QRS complexes are not preceded by P waves, but they are narrow so the rhythm is a junctional escape rhythm. The QRS duration is 94 ms, which is within normal limits.

Note the regular P waves marked with arrows. P waves are regular but have no clear relationship to the QRS complexes. This is called atrioventricular (AV) dissociation.

Note also the septal Q waves (leads V_2 and V_3) indicating possible previous myocardial infarction.

This is complete heart block or third degree AV block with AV dissociation.

The patient needs to be treated with the implantation of a permanent pacemaker unless a reversible cause is identified. Reversible causes include: AV node blocking agents such as beta-blockers, digoxin, verapamil, diltiazem; or metabolic abnormalities such as hyperkalaemia.

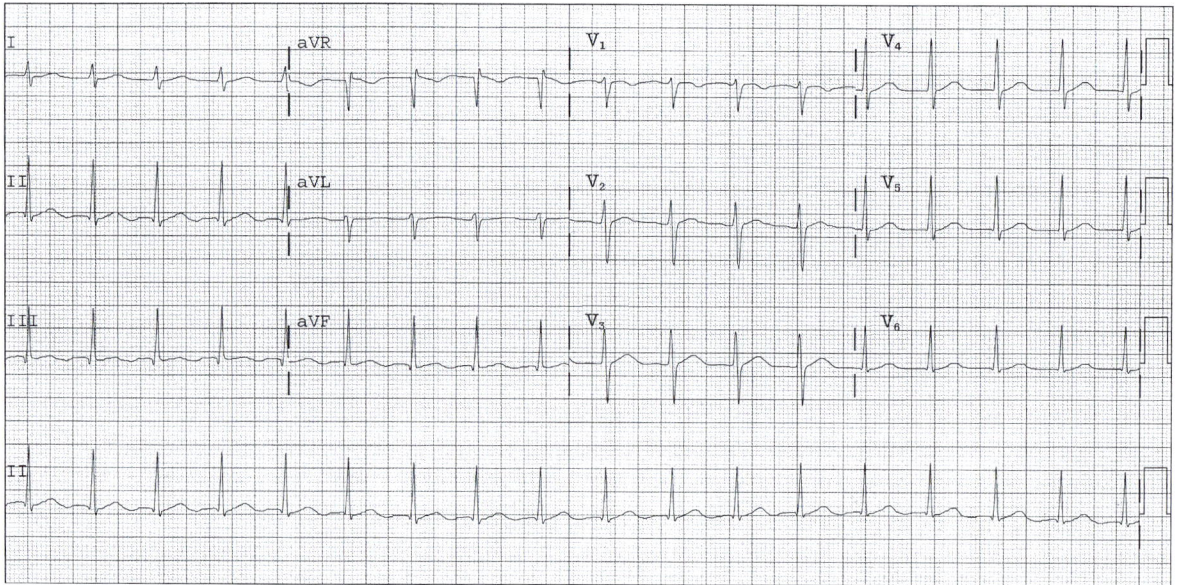

Figure 3.23a

CASE STUDY ON ECG 23

A 27-year-old woman presents with palpitations. She is otherwise well. Upon further assessment an ECG was obtained.

Please interpret the ECG in Figure 3.23a in a systematic manner.

Rhythm _____

Rate _____

Axis _____

P wave _____

PR interval _____

QRS complex _____

ST segment _____

T wave morphology _____

QT interval _____

Conclusion _____

Clinical notes _____

Diagnosis _____

_____

_____

_____

_____

Further investigations _____

_____

_____

_____

Management _____

_____

_____

_____

_____

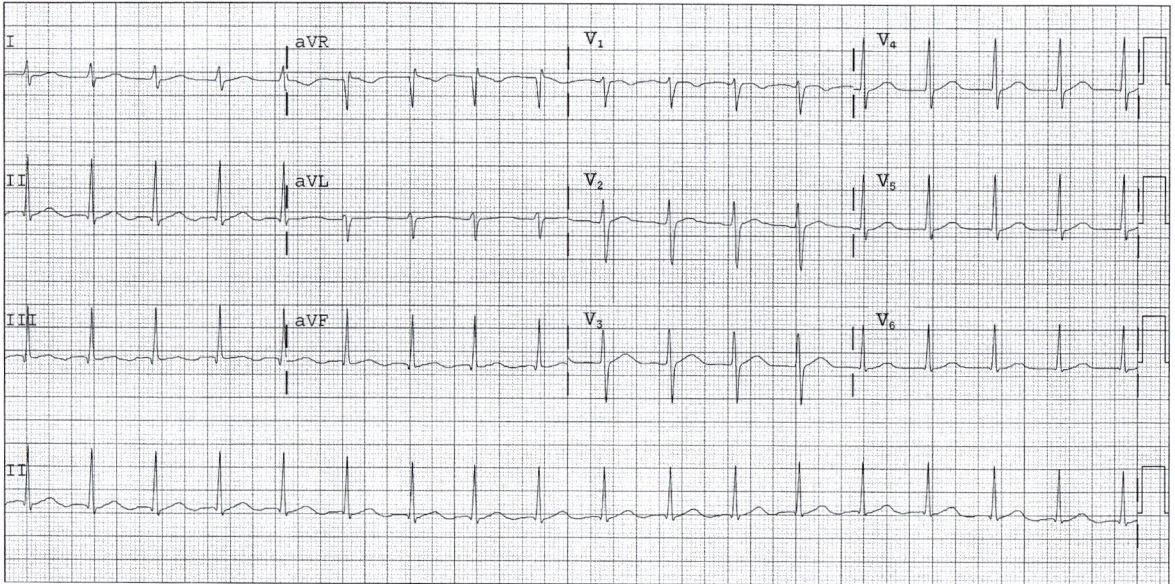

Figure 3.23b Junctional tachycardia

ANSWER TO CASE STUDY ON ECG 23: JUNCTIONAL TACHYCARDIA

A

Note that the rate is 110 bpm confirming tachycardia. Rhythm is regular (Fig 3.23b).

The QRS complex is narrow (85 ms) and not preceded by a P wave.

This is regular, narrow complex tachycardia in the absence of P waves, a junctional or AV nodal reentrant tachycardia. It is possible for retrograde P waves to be buried in the T waves, hence remaining not visible.

AV nodal reentrant tachycardia is the most common narrow complex tachycardia. More often this is seen in females, as is the case with this patient.

Vagal manoeuvres, such as carotid sinus massage or Valsalva manoeuvre, may increase the AV block and slow down the rate. Administration of adenosine too can bring about this effect. These measures may sometimes terminate the tachycardia, restoring sinus rhythm.

Sustained therapy requires AV nodal blocking agents such as beta-blockers, or calcium channel blockers such as verapamil or diltiazem.

The accessory reentry pathway can be ablated with radiofrequency energy upon electrophysiological study. This is indicated for those patients who are symptomatic and not responding to, or intolerant of, medical therapy. All above management steps are indicated in this patient.

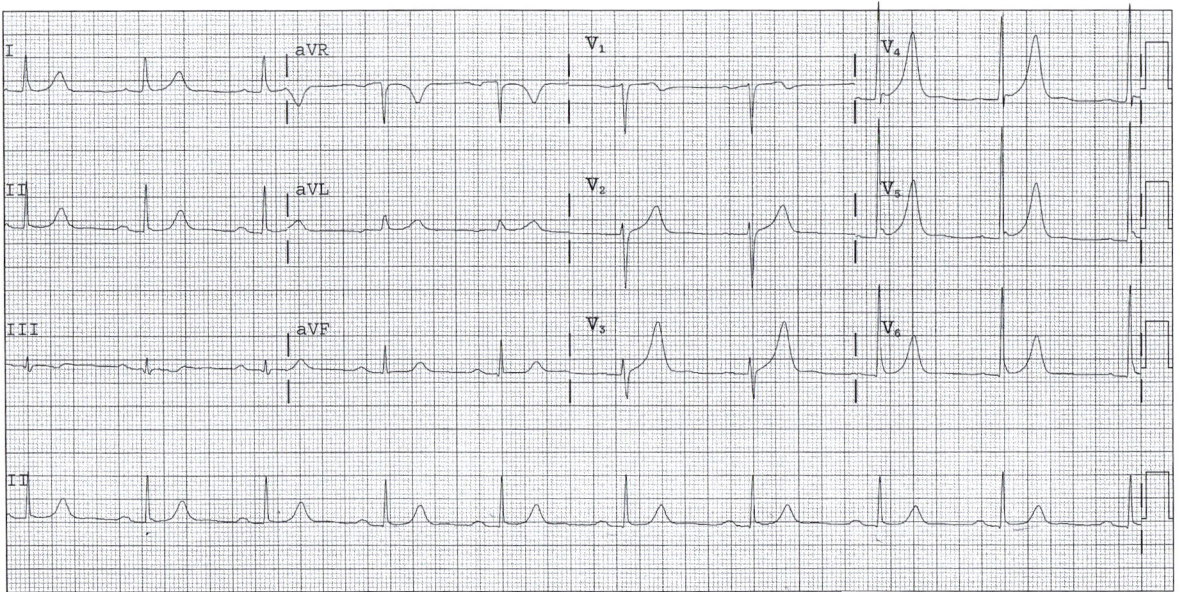

Figure 3.24a

CASE STUDY ON ECG 24

A 55-year-old man with chronic renal failure presents for dialysis. This ECG was taken pre-dialysis. He has chronic hypertension.

Please interpret the ECG in Figure 3.24a in a systematic manner.

Rhythm _____

Rate _____

Axis _____

P wave _____

PR interval _____

QRS complex _____

ST segment _____

T wave morphology _____

QT interval _____

Conclusion _____

Clinical notes _____

Diagnosis _____

_____

_____

_____

_____

Further investigations _____

_____

_____

_____

_____

Management _____

_____

_____

_____

_____

_____

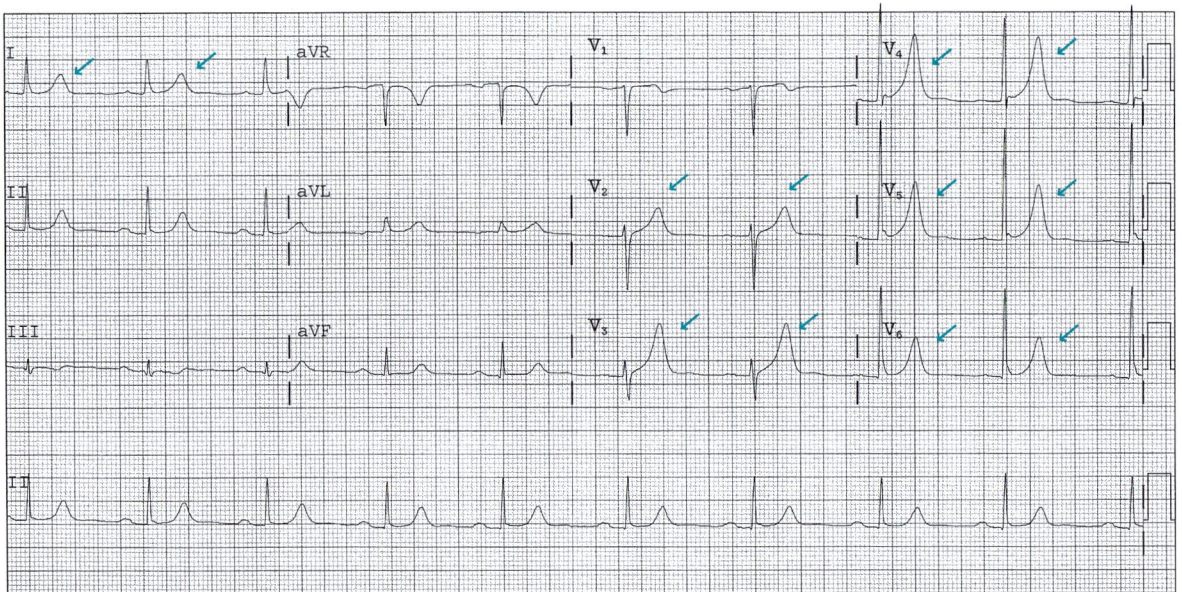

Figure 3.24b Hyperkalaemia

ANSWER TO CASE STUDY ON ECG 24: HYPERKALAEMIA

A

The rate is 56 bpm. Rhythm is regular. Axis is normal (Fig 3.24b).

PR interval is prolonged (marginally) indicating first degree heart block.

The most striking abnormality is the tall 'tented' T waves best seen in leads I, II, V_3, V_4, V_5 and V_6 (thin arrows). Also note that the P wave is very small in these leads.

These changes are usually due to hyperkalaemia in a patient who is dialysis dependent. His potassium (K^+) level is likely to be over 6 mmol/L.

When the serum K^+ level rises further, the PR interval is gradually prolonged leading to bradycardia and heart block.

The QRS complex will also widen and progress to a sinusoidal waveform. Eventually it will progress to ventricular tachycardia or ventricular fibrillation.

Treatment in this case is urgent dialysis to remove excess K^+ from the circulation.

The other therapeutic modalities for hyperkalaemia with cardiac manifestations include insulin–dextrose infusion, calcium chloride infusion and, if there is associated acidosis, bicarbonate infusion. This patient can be given a chelating agent such as resonium orally or per-rectally but this takes time to act. Stop any drugs that can cause hyperkalaemia such as ACE inhibitor, amiloride and spironolactone. Furosemide and salbutamol can also help reduce serum potassium levels.

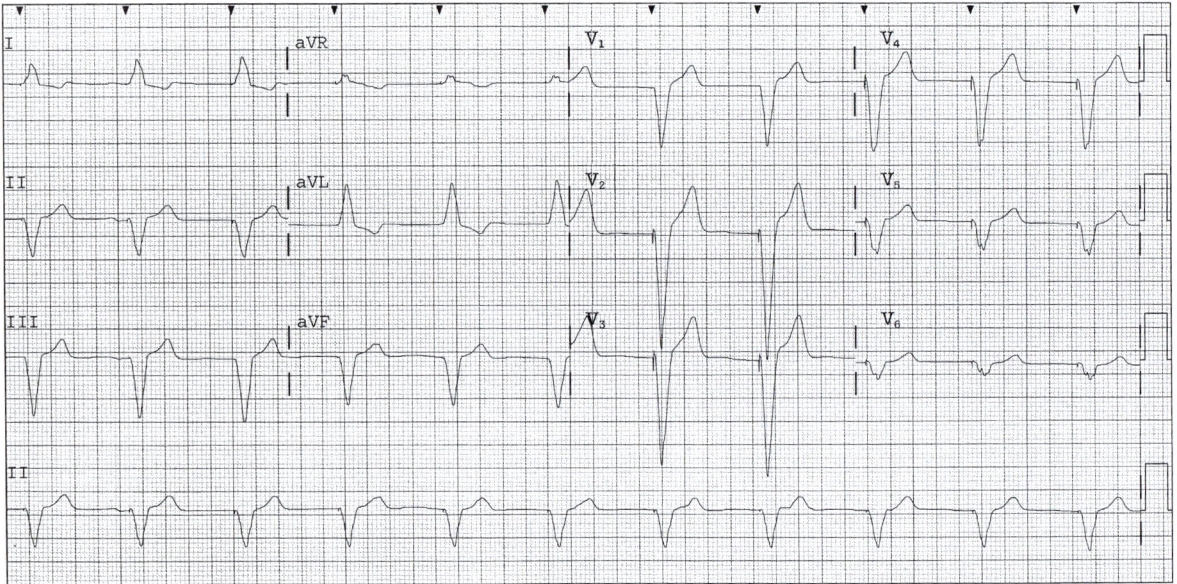

Figure 3.25a

CASE STUDY ON ECG 25

Q

This ECG was taken when an 86-year-old man presented for the investigation of dyspnoea.

Please interpret the ECG in Figure 3.25a in a systematic manner.

Rhythm _____

Rate _____

Axis _____

P wave _____

PR interval _____

QRS complex _____

ST segment _____

T wave morphology _____

QT interval _____

Conclusion _____

Clinical notes _____

Diagnosis _____

_____

_____

_____

_____

Further investigations _____

_____

_____

_____

_____

Management _____

_____

_____

_____

_____

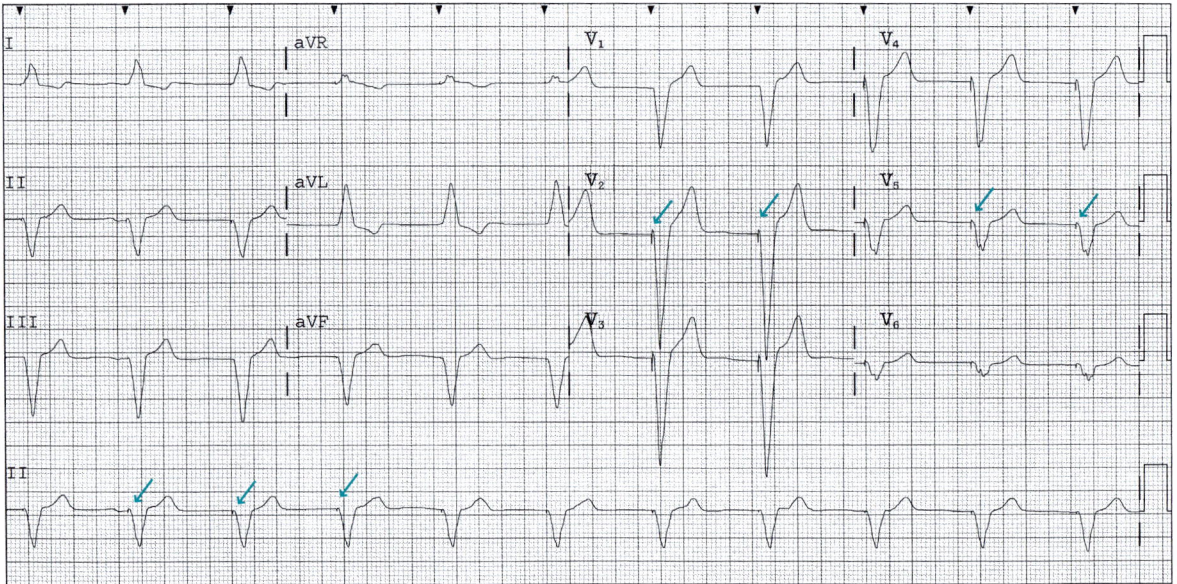

Figure 3.25b Paced rhythm (ventricular)

ANSWER TO CASE STUDY ON ECG 25: PACED RHYTHM (VENTRICULAR)

Note that the rate is 64 bpm and the rhythm is regular (Fig 3.25b). The axis is deviated to the left (−71°).

The QRS complex is broad (>120 ms). There are no P waves preceding the QRS complexes.

Note the pacing spikes as indicated by the arrows before the QRS complex. This together with the broad complex and the left bundle branch block pattern indicate that the patient's cardiac rhythm is generated by a ventricular pacemaker located in the right ventricle.

The lack of any atrial activity or an atrial-pacing spike indicates that only the ventricle is paced.

An LBBB pattern indicates that the right ventricle is depolarised before the left ventricle, as is the case when there is a true LBBB.

Paced rhythm cannot be used to interpret other cardiac pathology including coronary ischaemia.

The patient's heart is paced at a satisfactory rate. However pacemaker interrogation is indicated in the work-up to ensure that the rate response function is active. The rate response function enables the heart rate to be increased during exercise to ensure that the cardiac output is increased as required.

Pacemaker syndrome too should be considered as a differential diagnosis. The physiological synchrony with atrial contraction can be lost when the right ventricle alone is externally paced. This dis-synchrony between the atria and the ventricles can lead to irregularities in the diastolic filling of the ventricles and consequently to a reduction in the cardiac output. Some patients with pacemaker syndrome can present with dyspnoea. The treatment in this case would require referral to an electrophysiologist to place an additional lead in the left atrium. Once the left atrial lead is placed, the electrical pacing of the two chambers can be synchronised to mimic the natural rhythm thus restoring satisfactory cardiac output.

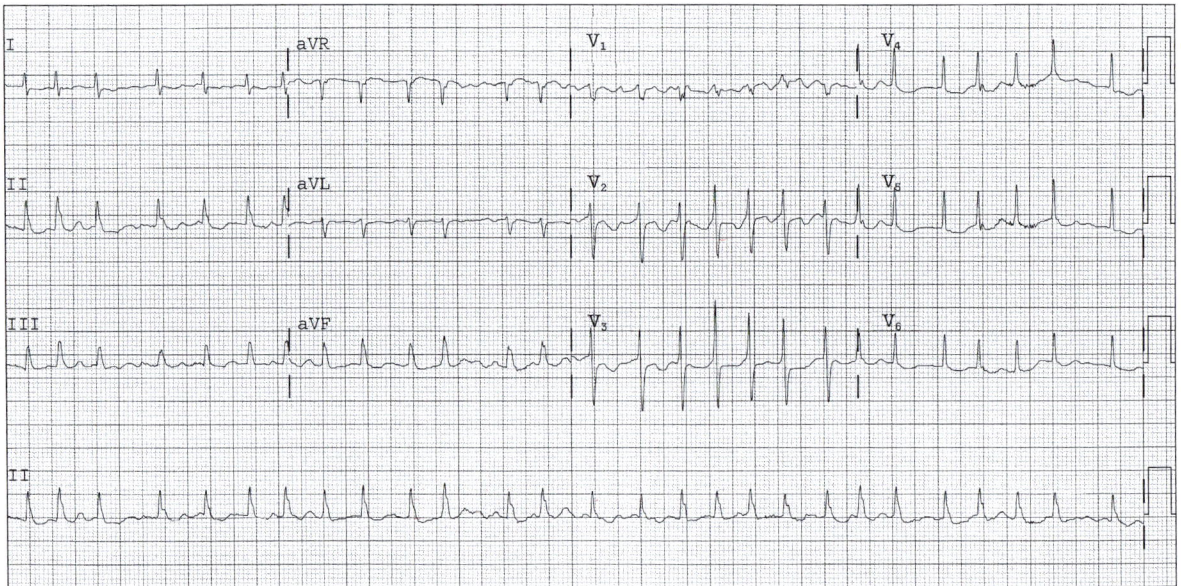

Figure 3.26a

CASE STUDY ON ECG 26

A 69-year-old woman presents with an ischaemic stroke. Upon further assessment an ECG was obtained.

Please interpret the ECG in Figure 3.26a in a systematic manner.

Rhythm _____

Rate _____

Axis _____

P wave _____

PR interval _____

QRS complex _____

ST segment _____

T wave morphology _____

QT interval _____

Conclusion _____

Clinical notes _____

Diagnosis _____

_____

_____

_____

_____

Further investigations _____

_____

_____

_____

_____

Management _____

_____

_____

_____

_____

_____

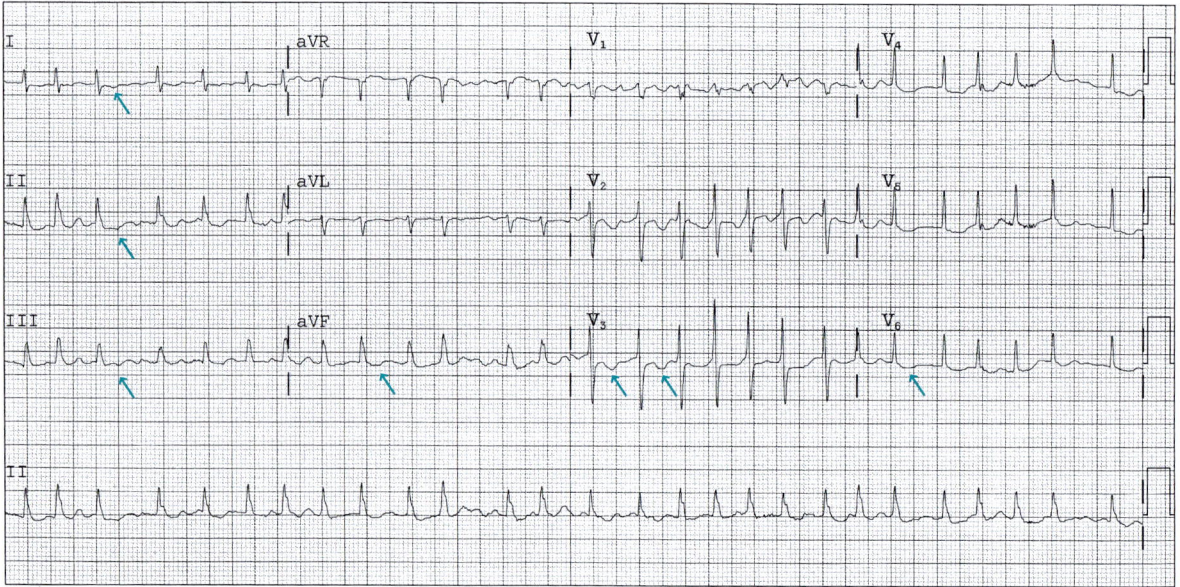

Figure 3.26b Atrial fibrillation

ANSWER TO CASE STUDY ON ECG 26: ATRIAL FIBRILLATION

A

Note that the rate is 170 bpm and the rhythm is irregularly irregular (Fig 3.26b). The axis is within normal limits but directed towards the right (88°). This is atrial fibrillation with a rapid ventricular response.

Note the diffuse T wave inversions seen in multiple leads (arrows). This may be due to coronary ischaemia induced by the patient's rapid ventricular rate.

The objectives of her management include stroke prevention, rate control or rhythm control, as required.

Rate control is the preferred strategy in this situation. It can be achieved with AV blocking agents such as digoxin, beta-blockers or non-dihydropyridine calcium channel blockers.

DC electrical cardioversion or an anti-arrhythmic agent such as amiodarone or sotalol can restore sinus rhythm.

Having had a stroke, this patient's risk of another embolic stroke is high (CHADS2 score is >2). She needs to be anticoagulated with warfarin or dabigatran if there is no significant risk of bleeding. A CT scan of the brain is indicated to rule out any intracranial bleeding or haemorrhagic transformation of the stroke before anticoagulation therapy.

Once her neurological status and AF have been stabilised, this patient needs further investigation to exclude underlying coronary ischaeamia. A dobutamine stress echocardiogram or a myocardial perfusion scan would be the initial non-invasive test in this case.

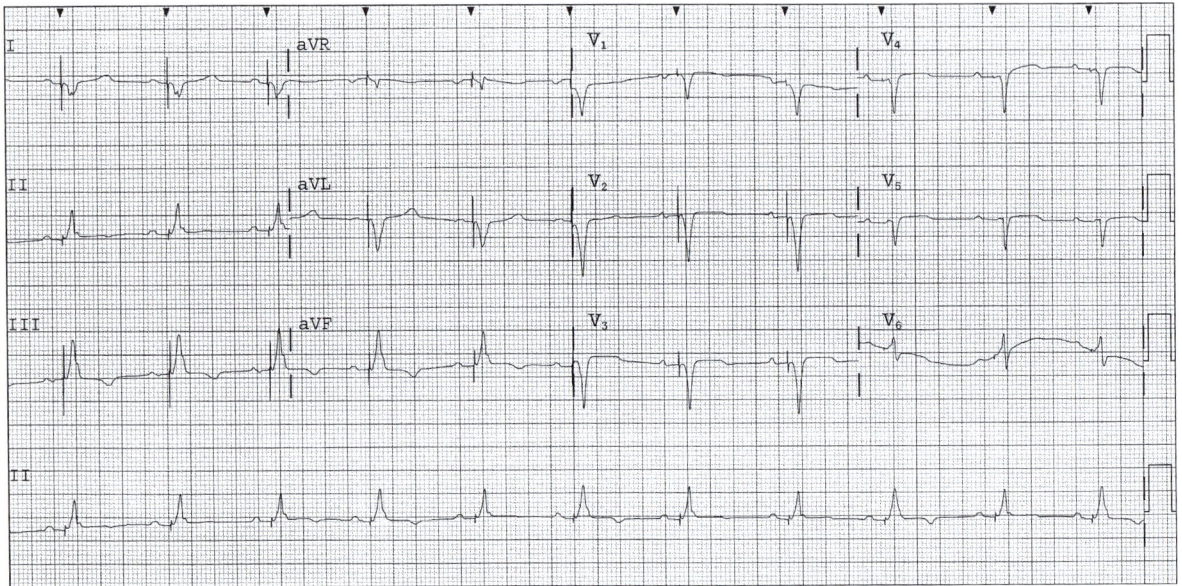

Figure 3.27a

CASE STUDY ON ECG 27

This 79-year-old patient was recently treated for recurrent syncope. Upon further assessment an ECG was obtained.

Please interpret the ECG in Figure 3.27a in a systematic manner.

Rhythm _____

Rate _____

Axis _____

P wave _____

PR interval _____

QRS complex _____

ST segment _____

T wave morphology _____

QT interval _____

Conclusion _____

Clinical notes _____

Diagnosis _____

_____

_____

_____

_____

Further investigations _____

_____

_____

_____

Management _____

_____

_____

_____

_____

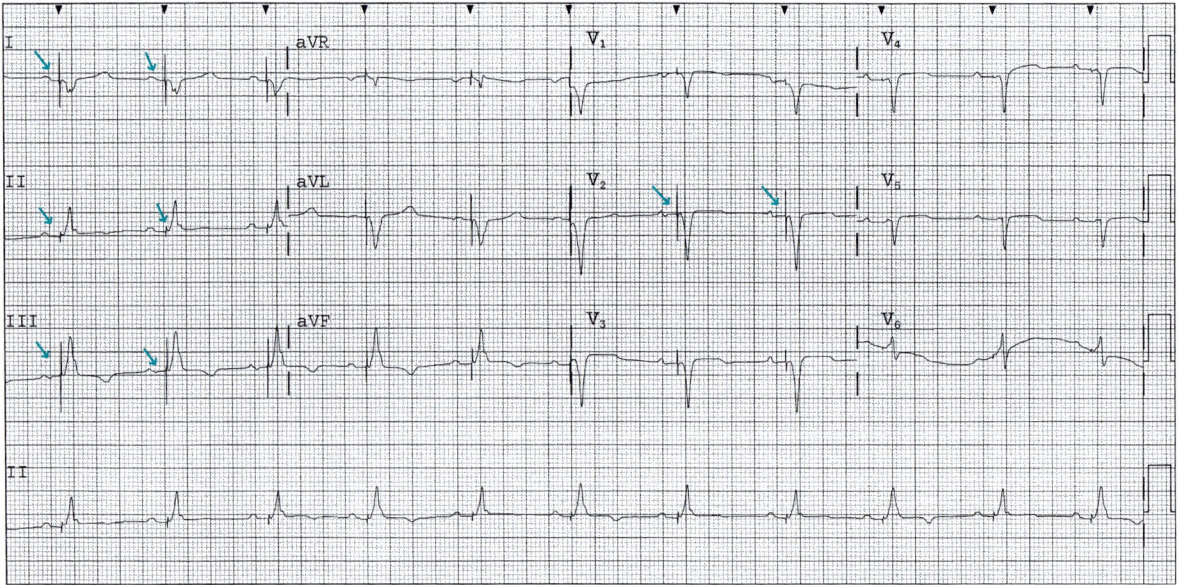

Figure 3.27b A sensed V-paced rhythm

ANSWER TO CASE STUDY ON ECG 27: A SENSED V-PACED RHYTHM

A

The rate is 66 bpm. The rhythm is regular (Fig 3.27b).

Note that there are regular P waves indicating sinus activity. Note the pacing spike (arrows) before each QRS complex that indicates ventricular pacing in the presence of preserved sinus activity in the atria. This patient has been treated with a ventricular pacemaker for complete heart block.

This ECG shows atrial sensed ventricular pacing where the pacemaker responds to the intrinsic sinoatrial node activity to time its impulse to the ventricle.

The possibility of complete heart block would explain his previous presentations with syncope. Now he has been treated with a ventricular pacemaker.

If he is asymptomatic since the pacemaker implantation he does not require further treatment.

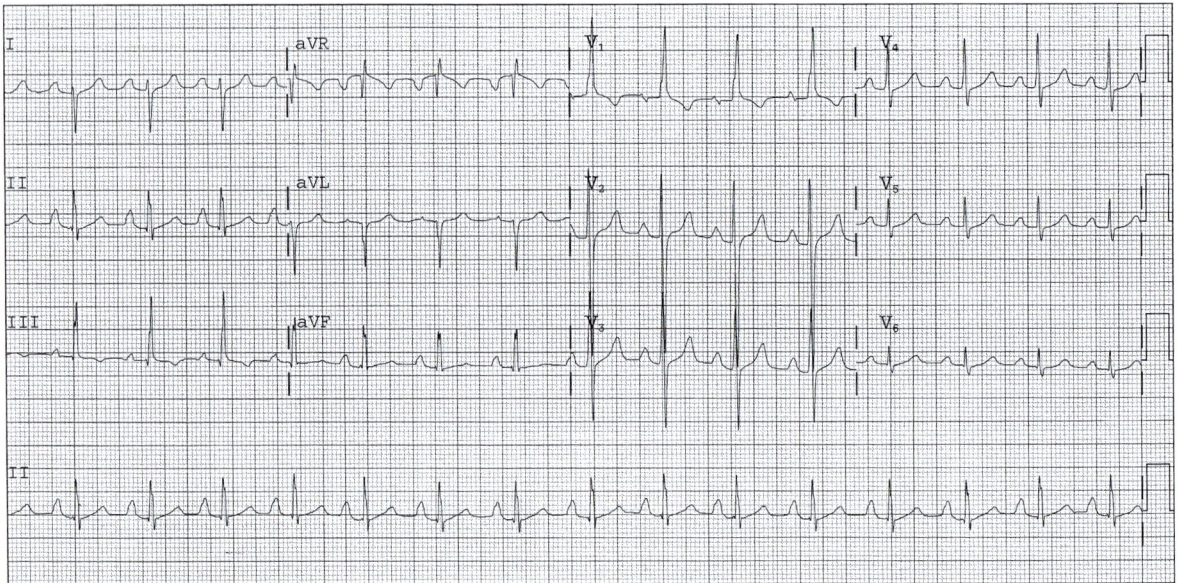

Figure 3.28a

CASE STUDY ON ECG 28

This 29-year-old female patient has a history of scleroderma. She now presents with progressive dyspnoea on exertion. Upon further assessment an ECG was obtained. Echocardiography in the past has revealed mild pulmonary hypertension.

Please interpret the ECG in Figure 3.28a in a systematic manner.

Rhythm _____

Rate _____

Axis _____

P wave _____

PR interval _____

QRS complex _____

ST segment _____

T wave morphology _____

QT interval _____

Conclusion _____

Clinical notes _____

Diagnosis _____

_____

_____

_____

_____

Further investigations _____

_____

_____

_____

_____

Management _____

_____

_____

_____

_____

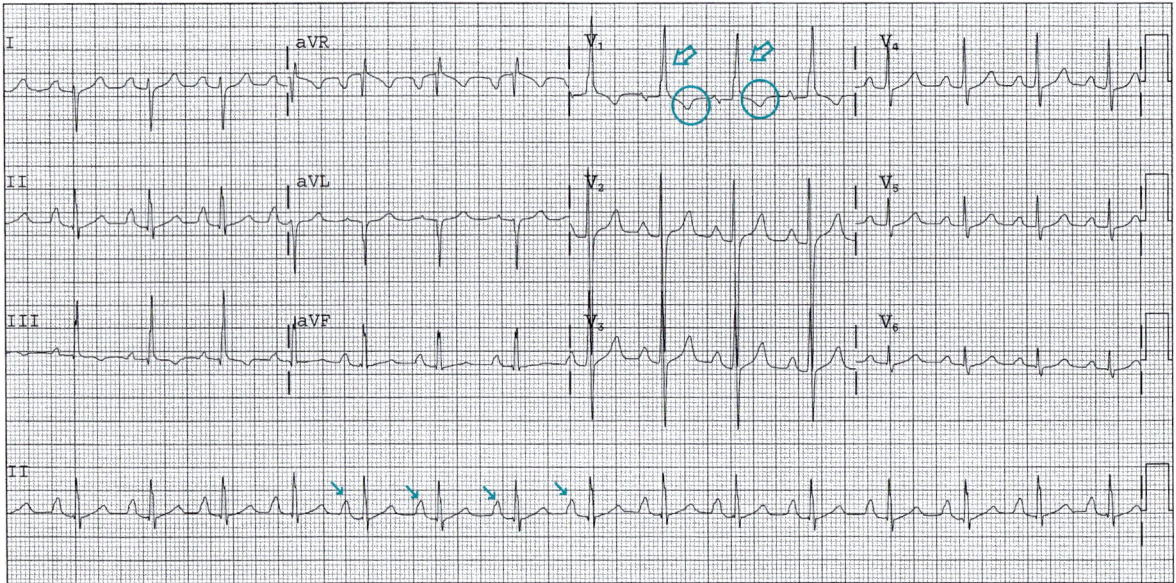

Figure 3.28b Right ventricular hypertrophy

ANSWER TO CASE STUDY ON ECG 28: RIGHT VENTRICULAR HYPERTROPHY

The rhythm is regular at a rate of 92 bpm. The axis is deviated to the right (Fig 3.28b).

One notable feature is the tall P wave that is best seen in lead II but evident in all leads (thin arrows). This is indicative of right atrial hypertrophy.

There are also features of right ventricular hypertrophy:

- Right axis deviation (axis deviated >100°)
- Tall R waves in lead V_1 (>6–7 mm) (thick arrows)
- T wave inversion in lead V_1.

Chronic pulmonary hypertension can lead to right ventricular hypertrophy. Pulmonary hypertension can also cause tricuspid regurgitation and right atrial hypertrophy over time. If untreated, chronic pulmonary arterial hypertension can lead to right heart failure. This is called cor pulmonale.

Examine her for any evidence of right heart failure such as elevated jugular venous pressure, painful hepatomegaly and peripheral oedema. Listen to the precordial region for a systolic murmur of tricuspid regurgitation.

This patient needs further investigations to establish the link between her presenting symptom of dyspnoea and pulmonary hypertension, which can be associated with scleroderma.

The next investigation to perform is an echocardiogram to check the right heart anatomy as well as pulmonary and right heart pressures. If the echocardiogram indicates the presence of significant pulmonary hypertension, she requires right heart catheterisation to confirm the diagnosis and to measure the pulmonary pressure accurately. If confirmed, she needs to be referred to a specialist physician with expertise in the management of pulmonary hypertension. She may require treatment for pulmonary hypertension with a designated agent, such as an endothelin-I receptor blocker or sildenafil, known to improve symptoms and prognosis.

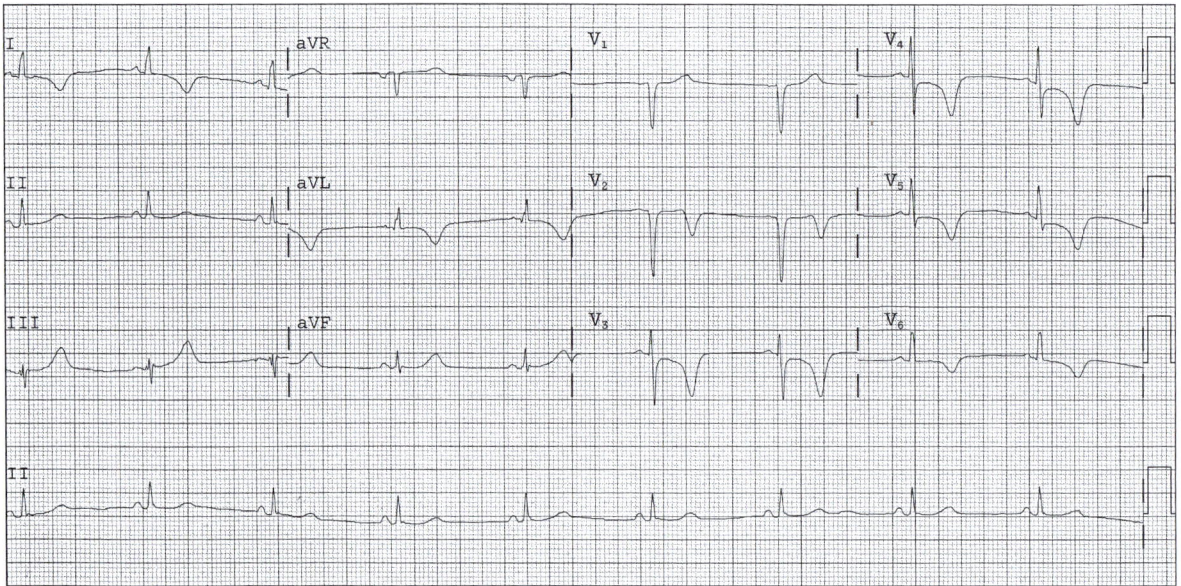

Figure 3.29a

CASE STUDY ON ECG 29

A 62-year-old male presents with severe retrosternal chest tightness, diaphoresis and dyspnoea. Upon further assessment an ECG was obtained.

Please interpret the ECG in Figure 3.29a in a systematic manner.

Rhythm _____

Rate _____

Axis _____

P wave _____

PR interval _____

QRS complex _____

ST segment _____

T wave morphology _____

QT interval _____

Conclusion _____

Clinical notes _____

Diagnosis _____

_____

_____

_____

_____

Further investigations _____

_____

_____

_____

Management _____

_____

_____

_____

_____

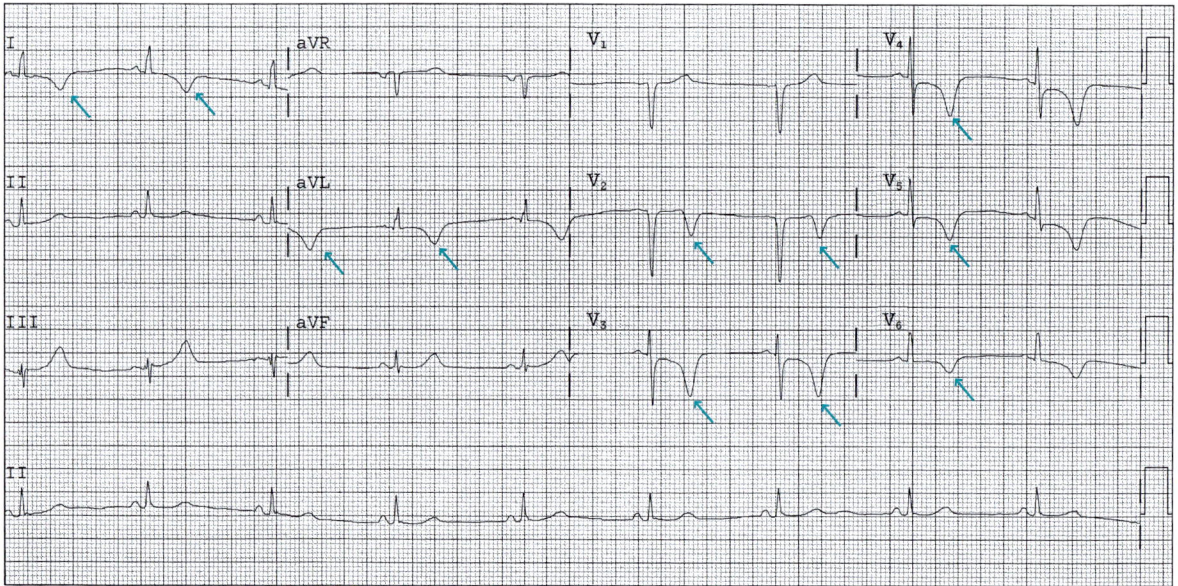

Figure 3.29b Acute coronary syndrome

ANSWER TO CASE STUDY ON ECG 29: ACUTE CORONARY SYNDROME

A

Note the rhythm is regular and the PR interval is short (120 ms). The axis is normal (Fig 3.29b).

The most striking abnormality is the T wave inversion seen in leads I, aVL, V_2, V_3, V_4, V_5 and V_6 (arrows). This is indicative of acute coronary ischaemia.

The diagnosis is acute coronary syndrome, unstable angina or non ST segment elevation infarction. The ECG changes suggest ischaemia of the lateral aspect of the left ventricle. It is therefore likely for the left circumflex artery or a large diagonal branch of the left anterior descending artery to be the vessel involved.

The patient needs to be urgently managed with antiplatelet therapy and anticoagulation to stabilise the ruptured plaque. Nitrates or morphine is needed to manage the pain. Cardiac troponin levels need to be checked and the patient needs to be closely monitored. Early catheterisation is indicated if the patient remains symptomatic or if serum troponin level is elevated.

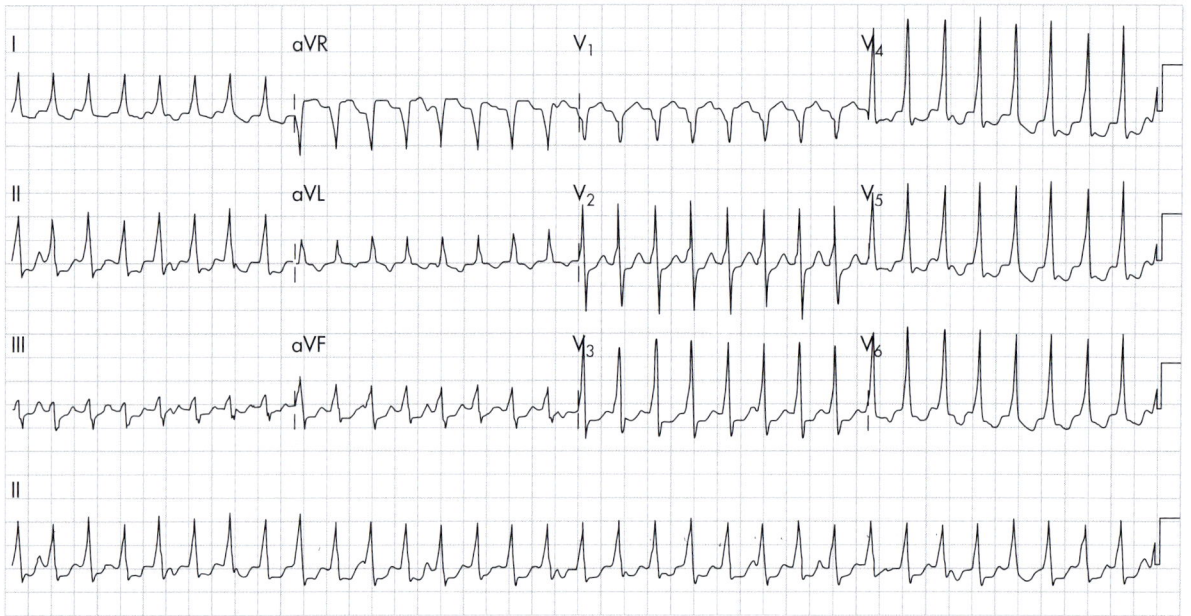

Figure 3.30a

CASE STUDY ON ECG 30

A 21-year-old woman presents with recurrent palpitations. She recalls losing consciousness in the past. Her blood pressure is 80/40 mmHg and she is complaining of feeling very light headed. Upon further assessment an ECG was obtained.

Please interpret the ECG in Figure 3.30a in a systematic manner.

Rhythm _____

Rate _____

Axis _____

P wave _____

PR interval _____

QRS complex _____

ST segment _____

T wave morphology _____

QT interval _____

Conclusion _____

Clinical notes _____

Diagnosis _____

_____

_____

_____

_____

Further investigations _____

_____

_____

_____

_____

Management _____

_____

_____

_____

_____

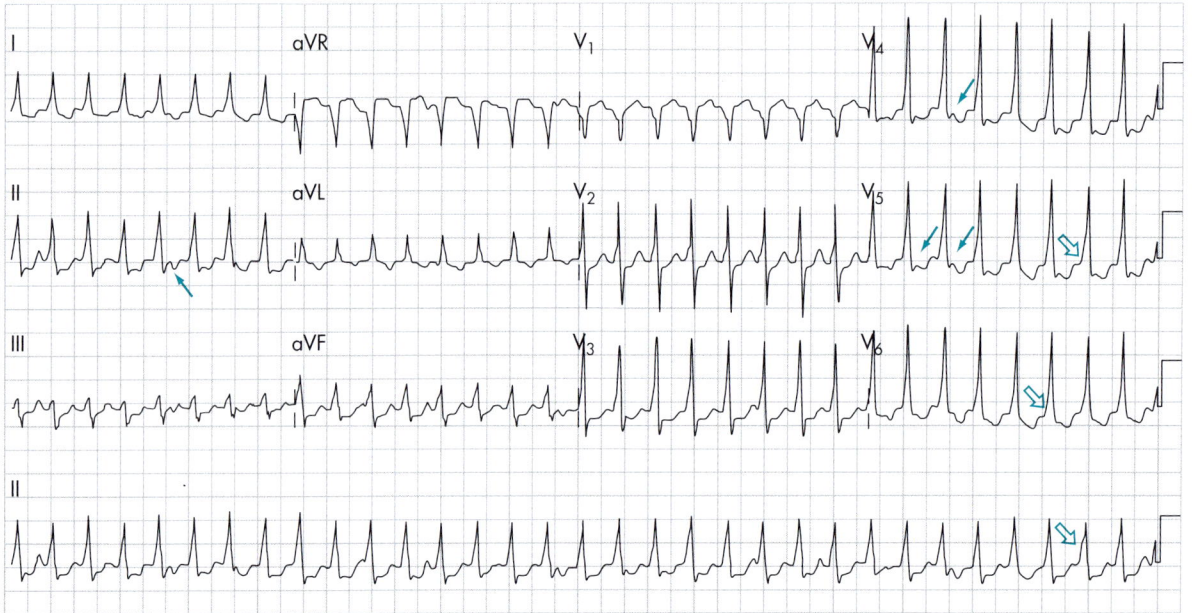

Figure 3.30b Wolff-Parkinson-White syndrome or supraventricular tachycardia

ANSWER TO CASE STUDY ON ECG 30: WOLFF-PARKINSON-WHITE SYNDROME OR SUPRAVENTRICULAR TACHYCARDIA

A

The rate is 200 bpm and the rhythm is regular (Fig 3.30b).

Retrograde P waves are clearly visible in some leads (thin arrows). Note that the P waves are inverted in the inferior lead, lead II.

QRS complexes are narrow but demonstrate a slurred upstroke, possibly a delta wave (thick arrows).

This is AV reentrant tachycardia due to an accessory pathway (bundle of Kent) indicating the diagnosis of Wolff-Parkinson-White syndrome.

The patient is haemodynamically unstable, hence she needs rapid induction of anaesthesia and urgent DC electrical cardioversion. Once sinus rhythm is restored her blood pressure should stabilise.

She needs definitive therapy with electrophysiological study and radiofrequency ablation of the accessory pathway given her past history of syncope and recurrent attacks.

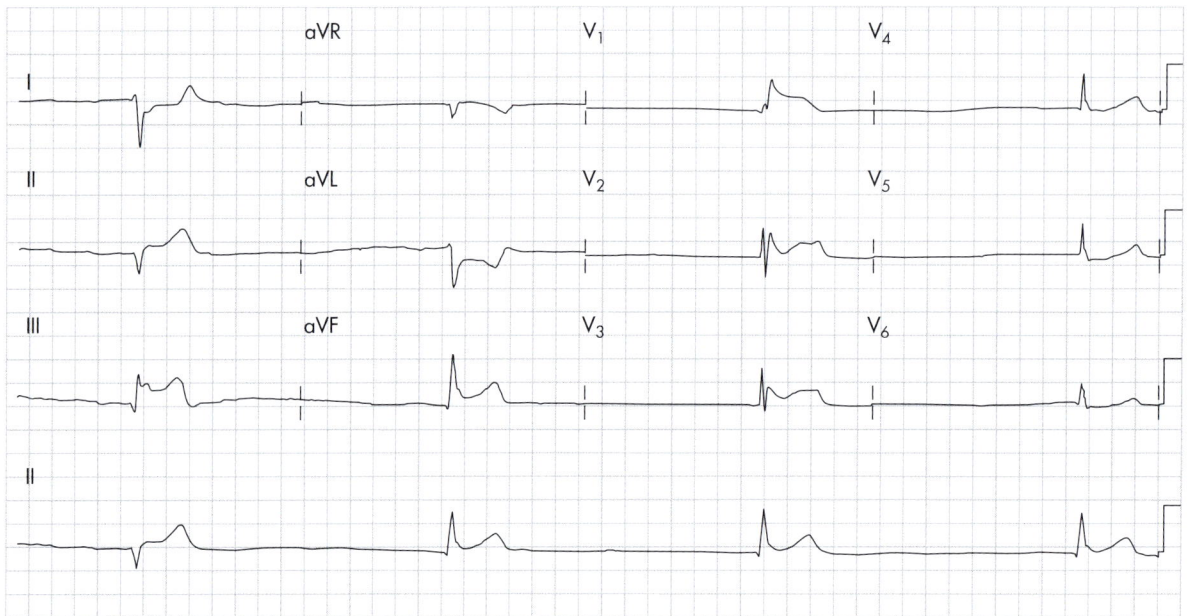

Figure 3.31a

CASE STUDY ON ECG 31

An 81-year-old woman presents with severe chest pain, nausea and vomiting. Upon presentation to the emergency department she loses consciousness. After further assessment an ECG was obtained.

Please interpret the ECG in Figure 3.31a in a systematic manner.

Rhythm _____

Rate _____

Axis _____

P wave _____

PR interval _____

QRS complex _____

ST segment _____

T wave morphology _____

QT interval _____

Conclusion _____

Clinical notes _____

Diagnosis _____

_____

_____

_____

_____

Further investigations _____

_____

_____

_____

Management _____

_____

_____

_____

_____

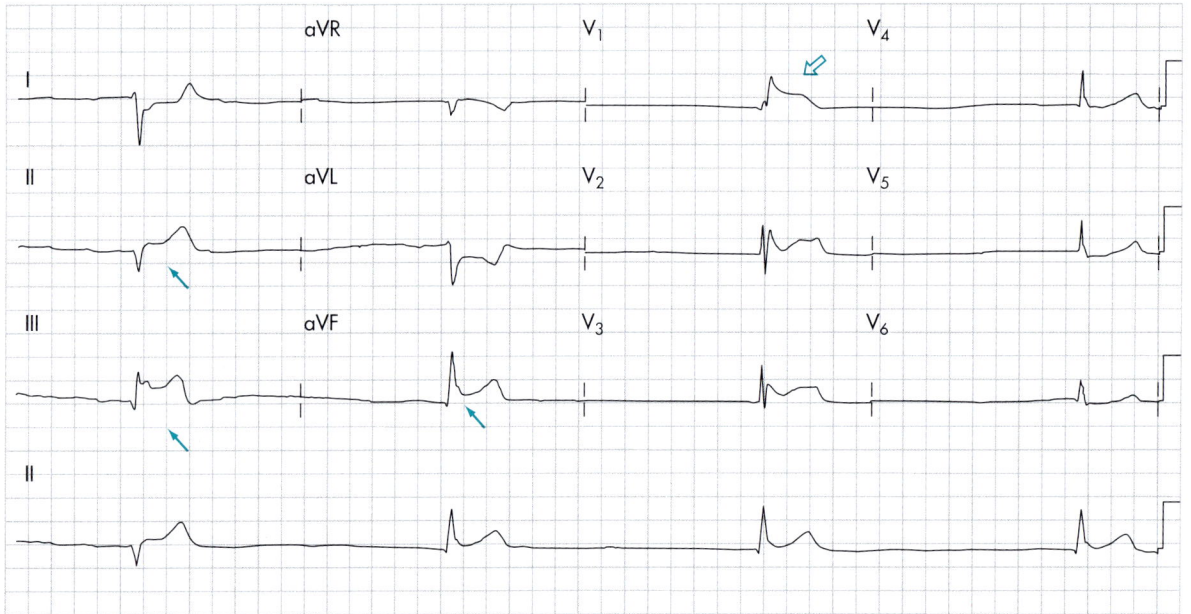

Figure 3.31b Right-sided STEMI

ANSWER TO CASE STUDY ON ECG 31: RIGHT-SIDED STEMI

A

Note the rate is 20 bpm. The rhythm is regular (Fig 3.31b).

She has no visible P waves. The QRS complexes are wide with RBBB morphology. She is in complete heart block with a ventricular escape rhythm.

Note the ST segment elevation in the inferior leads (leads II, III and aVF) (thin arrows). This indicates acute ischaemia and infarction of the inferior region of the left ventricle. This region is usually supplied by the right coronary artery.

There is ST segment elevation in V_1 (thick arrow) indicating the involvement of the right ventricle (RV). RV infarction is also signified by the relatively taller ST segment elevation in lead III compared to that of lead II.

The diagnosis of acute RV infarction can be confirmed by recording a right-sided ECG looking for ST segment elevation in the leads V_4R, V_5R and V_6R.

There are reciprocal changes in the lateral leads with ST segment depression seen in leads I and aVL.

This patient needs treatment with the immediate insertion of a temporary pacing wire into the right ventricle via the right femoral vein (while being stabilised by an external pacemaker). Coronary catheterisation is likely to show complete occlusion of the right coronary artery proximal to the origin of the right ventricular branch. This is the usual angiographic finding in the setting of acute RV infarction. The artery needs to be reopened with angioplasty and stent implantation. Restoration of blood supply to the affected region of the heart will lead to the restoration of sinus rhythm and stabilisation of blood pressure in many cases. Patients need copious fluid infusion to maintain blood pressure in the setting of RV infarction.

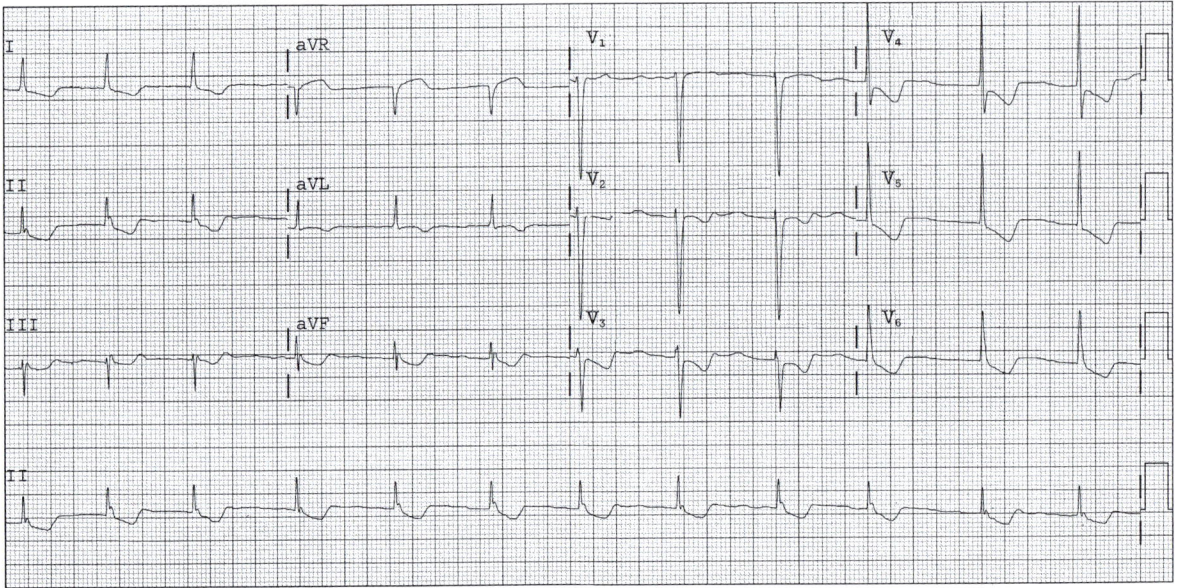

Figure 3.32a

CASE STUDY ON ECG 32

This 69-year-old woman presents with a two-day history of progressive nausea, vomiting and diarrhoea. She also complained of visual problems in the way of yellow-green halos. She has a history of paroxysmal atrial fibrillation and chronic renal failure. Her medication list includes digoxin 250 mcg per day and amiodarone 200 mcg per day. Upon further assessment an ECG was obtained.

Please interpret the ECG in Figure 3.32a in a systematic manner.

Rhythm _____

Rate _____

Axis _____

P wave _____

PR interval _____

QRS complex _____

ST segment _____

T wave morphology _____

QT interval _____

Conclusion _____

Clinical notes _____

Diagnosis _____

_____

_____

_____

_____

Further investigations _____

_____

_____

_____

_____

Management _____

_____

_____

_____

_____

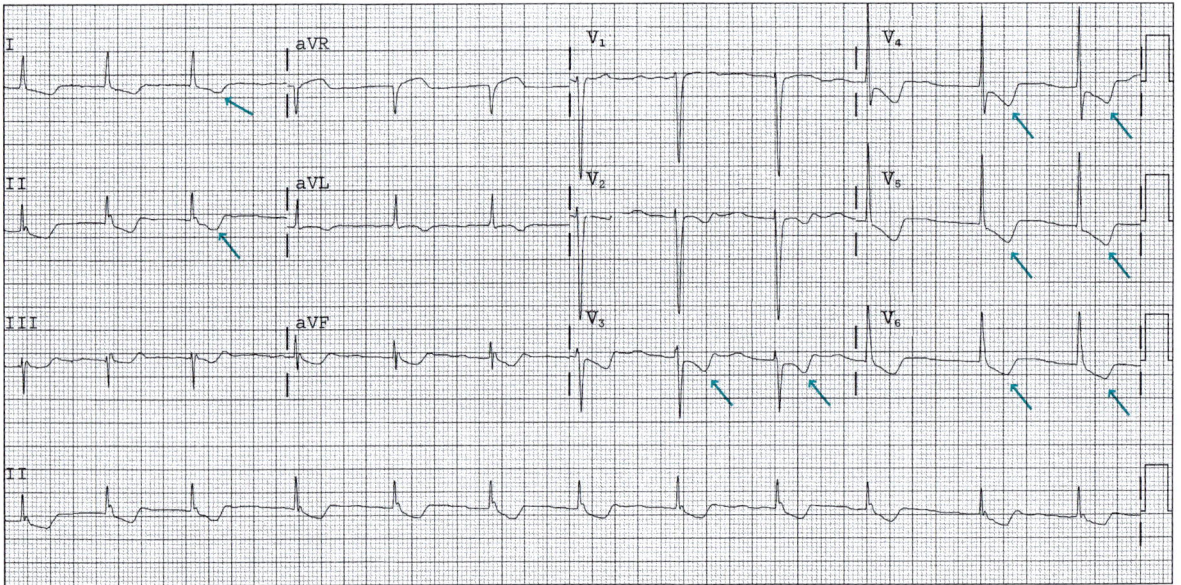

Figure 3.32b Digoxin toxicity

ANSWER TO CASE STUDY ON ECG 32: DIGOXIN TOXICITY

Note that the rhythm is irregularly irregular with a ventricular rate of 71 bpm (Fig 3.32b).

The most notable features are the ST depression and T wave inversion seen in leads I, II, V_3, V_4, V_5 and V_6 (arrows). This T wave inversion has the shape of a 'reverse tick', which is characteristic of digoxin toxicity. Blood should be tested for digoxin level, which is likely to be in the toxic range.

Digoxin effect (not toxicity) on ECG is manifested as ST depression and T wave inversion. Digoxin toxicity will make these changes more marked. In digoxin toxicity you may also see:

- Prolongation of the PR interval
- Bradycardia that can progress to heart block
- Shortening of the QT interval
- Ventricular ectopic beats, bigeminy
- Ventricular tachycardia, ventricular fibrillation.

Clinical features of digoxin toxicity include:

- Lethargy, nausea, vomiting and diarrhoea
- Syncope
- Palpitations, chest pain and dyspnoea
- Headache and acute confusion
- Yellow-green vision, halos, blurred vision, diplopia.

Digoxin toxicity should be managed with the immediate withdrawal of the agent and also cessation of any other medication that can precipitate digoxin toxicity, such as amiodarone, verapamil or erythromycin. The patient should be hydrated well. If conservative measures fail to relieve symptoms and/or if cardiac manifestations are present, the patient should be given antibody fragments against digoxin (digibind). Severe bradycardia with hypotension may require the insertion of a temporary pacemaker.

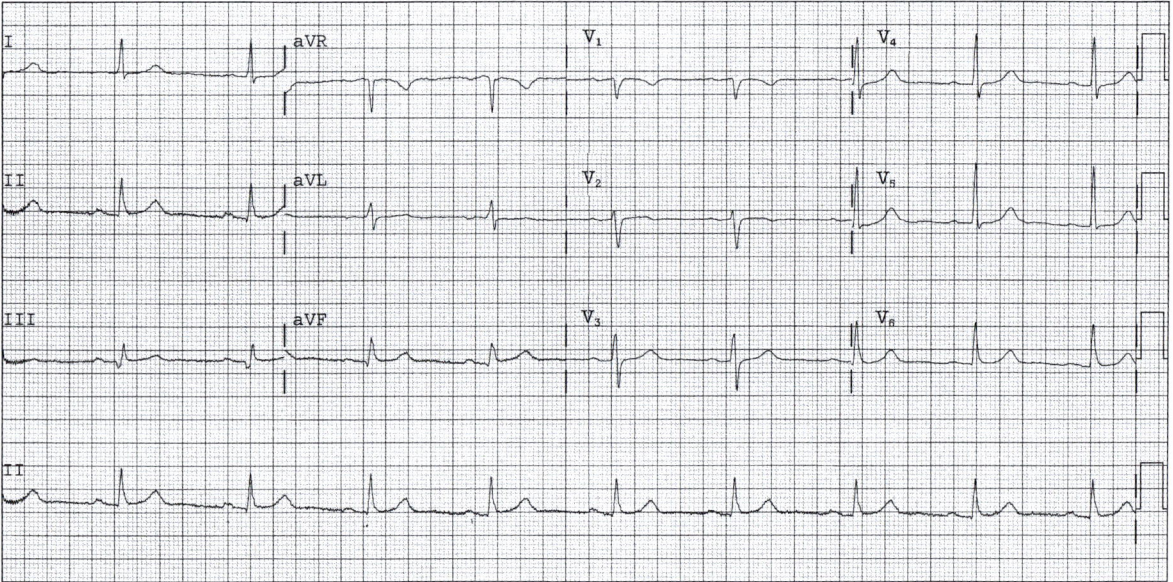

Figure 3.33a

CASE STUDY ON ECG 33

A 21-year-old woman presents with retrosternal chest tightness. She denies any pleuritic features to her chest pain. She has no past history of cardiac disease, and no known cardiovascular risk factors. Upon further assessment an ECG was obtained.

Please interpret the ECG in Figure 3.33a in a systematic manner.

Rhythm _____

Rate _____

Axis _____

P wave _____

PR interval _____

QRS complex _____

ST segment _____

T wave morphology _____

QT interval _____

Conclusion _____

Clinical notes _____

Diagnosis _____

_____

_____

_____

_____

Further investigations _____

_____

_____

_____

_____

Management _____

_____

_____

_____

_____

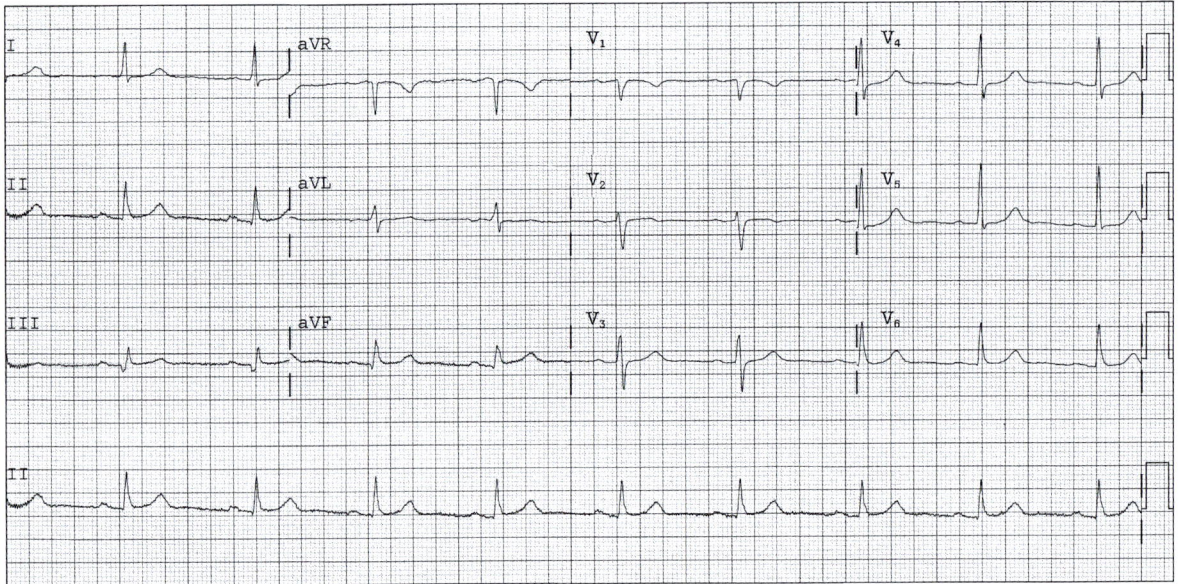

Figure 3.33b Normal

ANSWER TO CASE STUDY ON ECG 33: NORMAL

A

The rhythm is regular and each QRS complex is preceded by a P wave, hence it is sinus rhythm (Fig 3.33b).

The PR interval is 200 ms and normal. The QRS axis is normal at 41°. The QRS complex is of normal duration (110 ms) and there is no evidence of abnormalities such as Q waves. The ST segment remains within the baseline with no shifting. T wave is upright and within normal parameters. QT interval too is normal at 449 ms.

This ECG is a normal ECG. It is important to be very familiar with a normal ECG to be able to spot abnormalities accurately and rapidly.

Given the symptom of chest pain, you should look for any changes that could suggest coronary ischaemia (ST segment shift or T wave inversion) or pericarditis (ST segment elevation of concave-up morphology). None is seen in this ECG.

However a careful physical examination is indicated to look for other causes of chest pain. Tenderness in the costochondral region may suggest costochondritis that can be managed with a trial of an antiinflammatory agent. Tenderness in the epigastric region may suggest a gastric pathology. A positive Murphy's sign may suggest cholelithiasis.

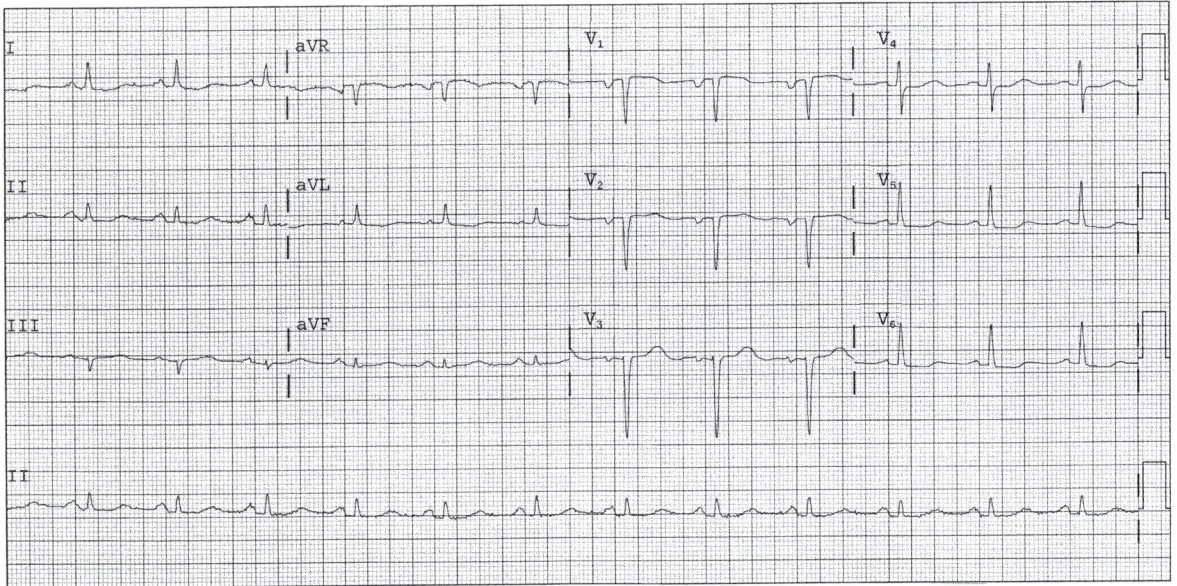

Figure 3.34a

CASE STUDY ON ECG 34

Q

A 45-year-old Indigenous woman presents with acute pulmonary oedema. She is a smoker. Her past medical history includes rheumatic fever in childhood. Close examination revealed an opening snap and a mid-diastolic murmur of mitral stenosis. Upon further assessment an ECG was obtained.

Please interpret the ECG in Figure 3.34a in a systematic manner.

Rhythm _____

Rate _____

Axis _____

P wave _____

PR interval _____

QRS complex _____

ST segment _____

T wave morphology _____

QT interval _____

Conclusion _____

Clinical notes _____

Diagnosis _____

_____

_____

_____

_____

Further investigations _____

_____

_____

_____

_____

Management _____

_____

_____

_____

_____

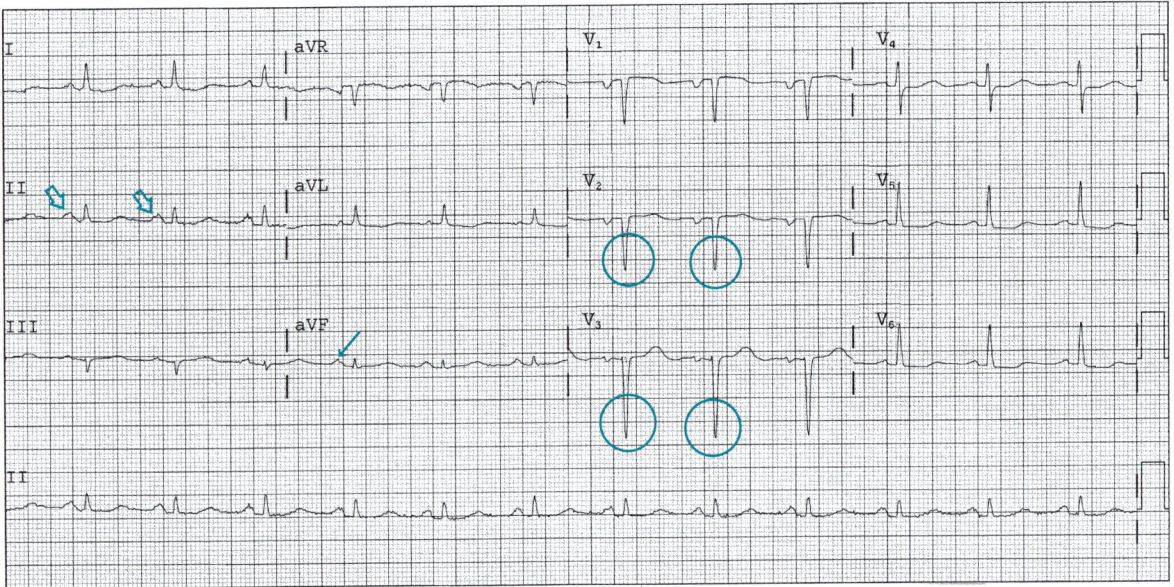

Figure 3.34b Septal Q waves

ANSWER TO CASE STUDY ON ECG 34: SEPTAL Q WAVES

Note that this patient is in sinus rhythm. The rate is 75 bpm. Axis is within normal limits (Fig 3.34b).

The most relevant finding to the presenting symptom is the significant Q wave seen in leads V_2 and V_3 (circles). This is indicative of previous myocardial infarction in the septal region of the left ventricle. She also has T wave inversion in leads I and aVL, and it is biphasic or flattened in leads V_5 and V_6. This is indicative of acute coronary ischaemia. Immediately check her serum troponin levels.

Note that the P wave in lead II is prolonged at 160 ms (normal is <120 ms) (thick arrows). It is notched in lead aVF (thin arrow). This is indicative of left atrial hypertrophy (also called p mitrale). These findings complement the clinical picture of rheumatic fever in the past and subsequent mitral stenosis (as suggested by the diastolic murmur). Chronic mitral stenosis can lead to left atrial hypertrophy.

The absolute clinical priority is to treat the pulmonary oedema and precipitating coronary ischaemia. An urgent chest X-ray is indicated to confirm the diagnosis and also to assess the severity of pulmonary congestion. She needs to be stabilised with intravenous diuretic therapy, intravenous nitrate therapy and intravenous morphine therapy. Her oxygenation should be supported with 100 per cent oxygen supplementation via the non-rebreather mask. Her serum cardiac troponin level needs to be tested for myocardial injury, which could precipitate acute heart failure. She needs anticoagulation and antiplatelet therapy. Once her pulmonary oedema is treated she may benefit from cardiac catheterisation for coronary revascularisation.

She needs an echocardiogram to assess her left ventricular anatomy and function. This will also give information about her left atrium and mitral valve. Mitral stenosis can be treated with balloon valvuloplasty or surgical repair or replacement as indicated by the severity of the lesion.

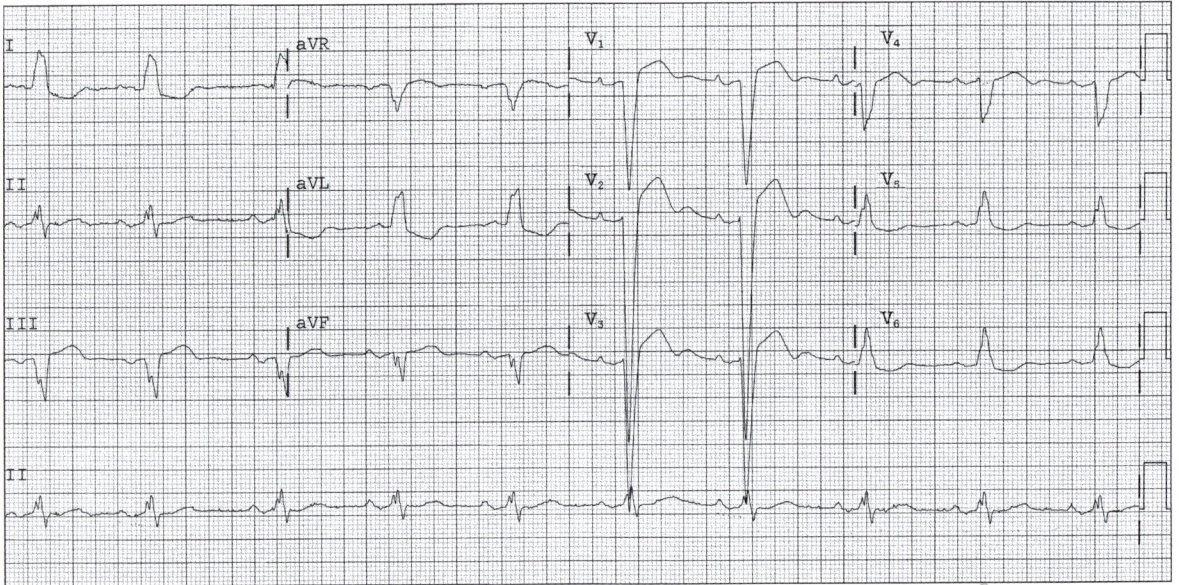

Figure 3.35a

CASE STUDY ON ECG 35

A 55-year-old male smoker presents with severe chest tightness that radiated to the left jaw. Previous ECG tracings in his medical records were all normal. The patient was in severe distress at presentation. Upon further assessment an ECG was obtained.

Please interpret the ECG in Figure 3.35a in a systematic manner.

Rhythm _____

Rate _____

Axis _____

P wave _____

PR interval _____

QRS complex _____

ST segment _____

T wave morphology _____

QT interval _____

Conclusion _____

Clinical notes _____

Diagnosis _____

_____

_____

_____

_____

Further investigations _____

_____

_____

_____

Management _____

_____

_____

_____

_____

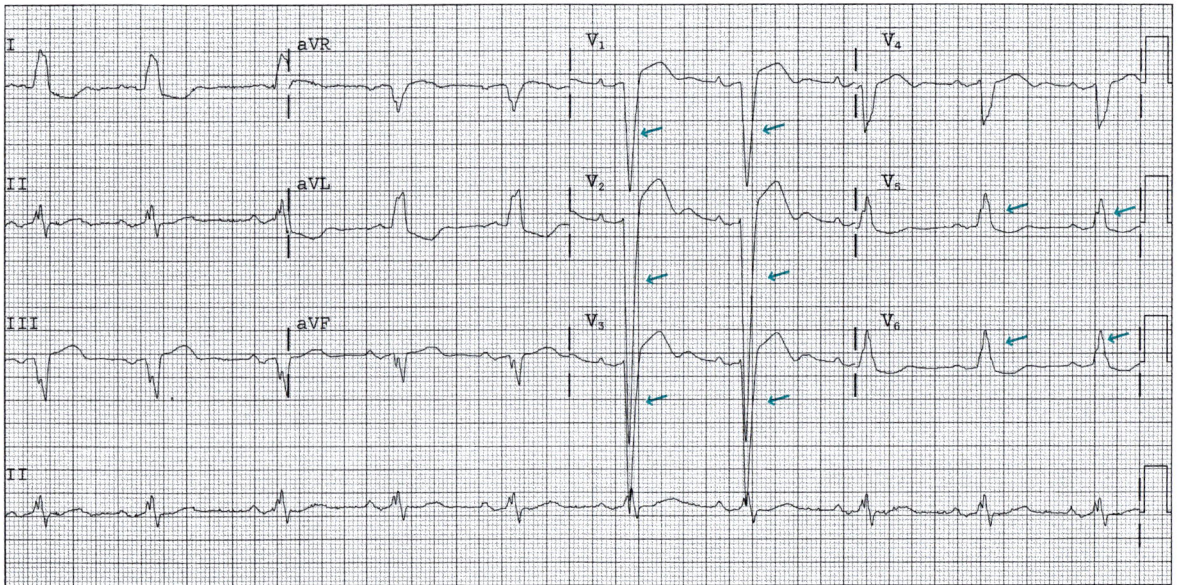

Figure 3.35b Left axis deviation and LBBB

ANSWER TO CASE STUDY ON ECG 35: LEFT AXIS DEVIATION AND LBBB

A

The rhythm is regular and sinus in origin. The rate is 60 bpm. The axis is shifted to the left (Fig 3.35b).

Note the QRS complex is wide (>120 ms) with a left bundle branch block pattern seen in the precordial leads (thin arrows).

The features of LBBB include:

- Prominent and wide R waves in leads V_5, V_6, aVL and I
- Prominent S wave or QS complex in lead V_1
- Poor R wave progression in leads V_1 to V_3
- ST segment depression in leads V_5 and V_6, together with T wave inversion and ST segment elevation in leads V_1, V_2 and V_3 (discordant ST segment shift).

Note also the ST segment elevation seen in lead III. This is not complemented with similar ST segment elevation in leads II and aVF.

Given that his previous ECG tracings were normal, it is clear that the LBBB is new. A diagnosis of acute myocardial infarction should be made with the patient referred to the interventional cardiology team for immediate cardiac catheterisation and primary angioplasty. If a primary angioplasty service is not available the patient needs thrombolysis, unless contraindicated.

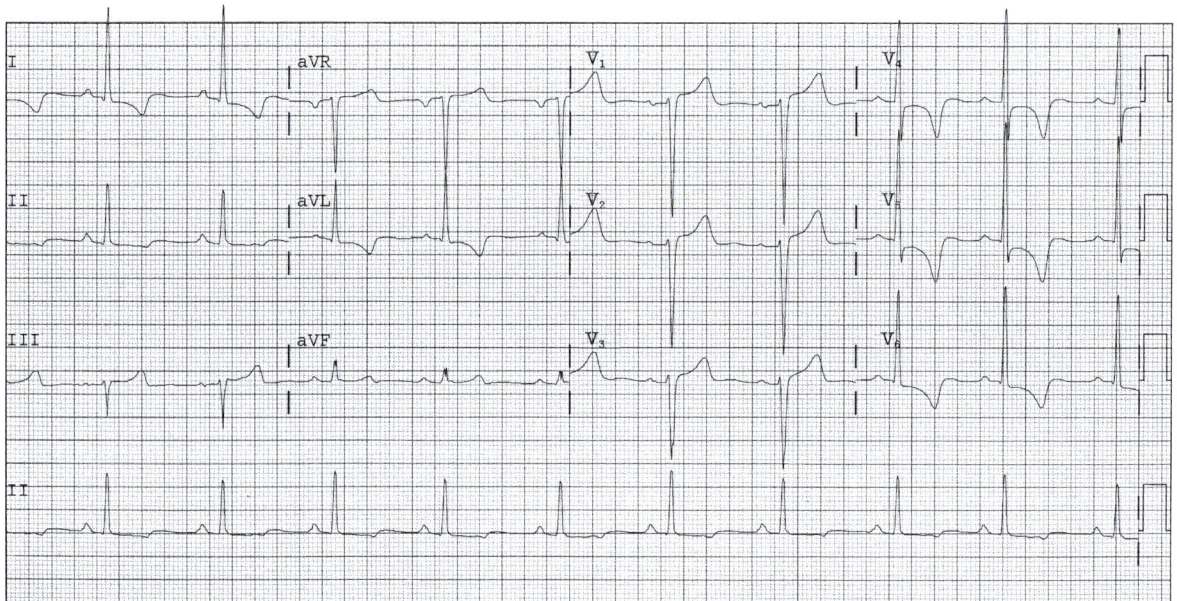

Figure 3.36a

CASE STUDY ON ECG 36

This 40-year-old female presents with two episodes of syncope. On examination she had a loud systolic murmur and a precordial heave. The patient was normotensive with no past history of hypertension. Upon further assessment an ECG was obtained.

Please interpret the ECG in Figure 3.36a in a systematic manner.

Rhythm _____

Rate _____

Axis _____

P wave _____

PR interval _____

QRS complex _____

ST segment _____

T wave morphology _____

QT interval _____

Conclusion _____

Clinical notes _____

Diagnosis _____

_____

_____

_____

_____

Further investigations _____

_____

_____

_____

Management _____

_____

_____

_____

_____

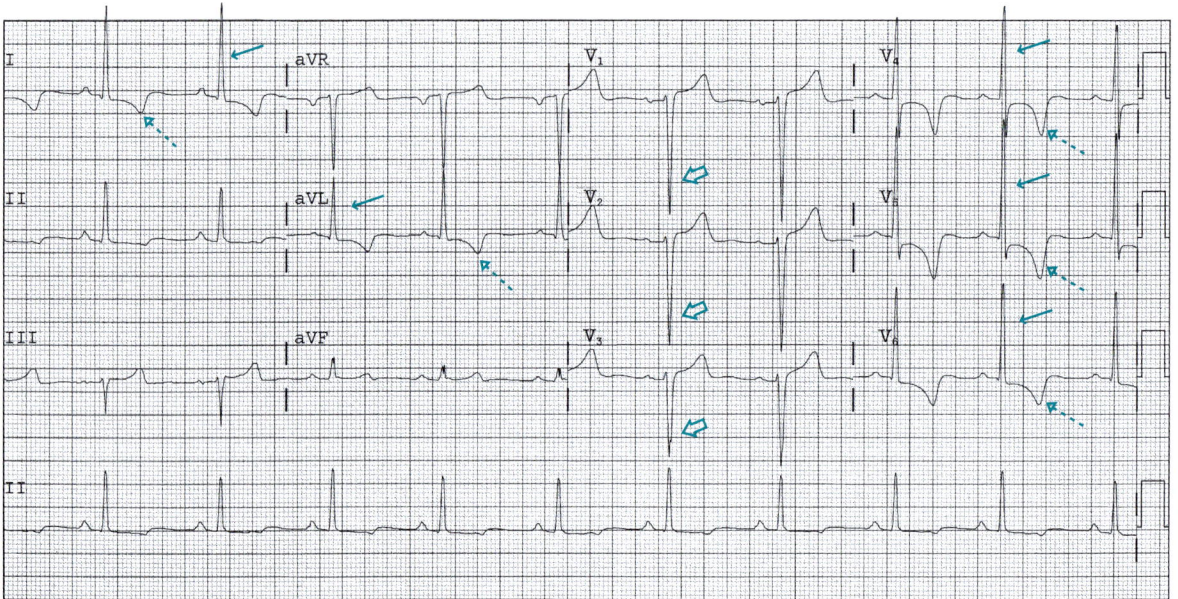

Figure 3.36b Left ventricular hypertrophy and HOCM

ANSWER TO CASE STUDY ON ECG 36: LEFT VENTRICULAR HYPERTROPHY AND HOCM

A

The rhythm is sinus at a rate of 60 bpm. The axis is within normal limits (Fig 3.36b).

The most striking abnormalities in the ECG are the deep S waves seen in leads V_1, V_2 and V_3 (thick arrows) and tall R waves seen in leads V_4, V_5 and V_6. R waves are tall in the leads I and aVL too (thin arrows). These findings are highly indicative of left ventricular hypertrophy (LVH).

The T wave inversion and ST segment depression seen in the leads V_4, V_5, V_6, I and aVL indicate repolarisation effects of LVH (broken arrows).

In the absence of hypertension and with a history of syncope, hypertrophic obstructive cardiomyopathy or severe aortic stenosis should be suspected. Severe aortic stenosis is rather uncommon in this age group. It is seen mostly in the elderly.

The patient needs further investigation with echocardiography looking for aortic stenosis or hypertrophic obstructive cardiomyopathy (HOCM) with asymmetric septal hypertrophy (septum is significantly thicker than the left ventricular free wall). The latter is the more likely diagnosis in this case. Another feature of HOCM is the anterior motion of the anterior leaflet of the mitral valve during systole. This movement of the valve leaflet can obstruct the left ventricular outflow tract. This phenomenon is called systolic anterior motion (SAM) of the mitral valve. In HOCM the pressure gradient across the left ventricular outflow tract (LVOT) is usually high indicating obstruction to blood flow out of the heart. If present this finding could explains her syncope.

She needs to be commenced on a beta-blocker in the first instance. If this therapy does not help reduce the LVOT gradient she may require alcohol septal ablation or surgical reduction of the septum.

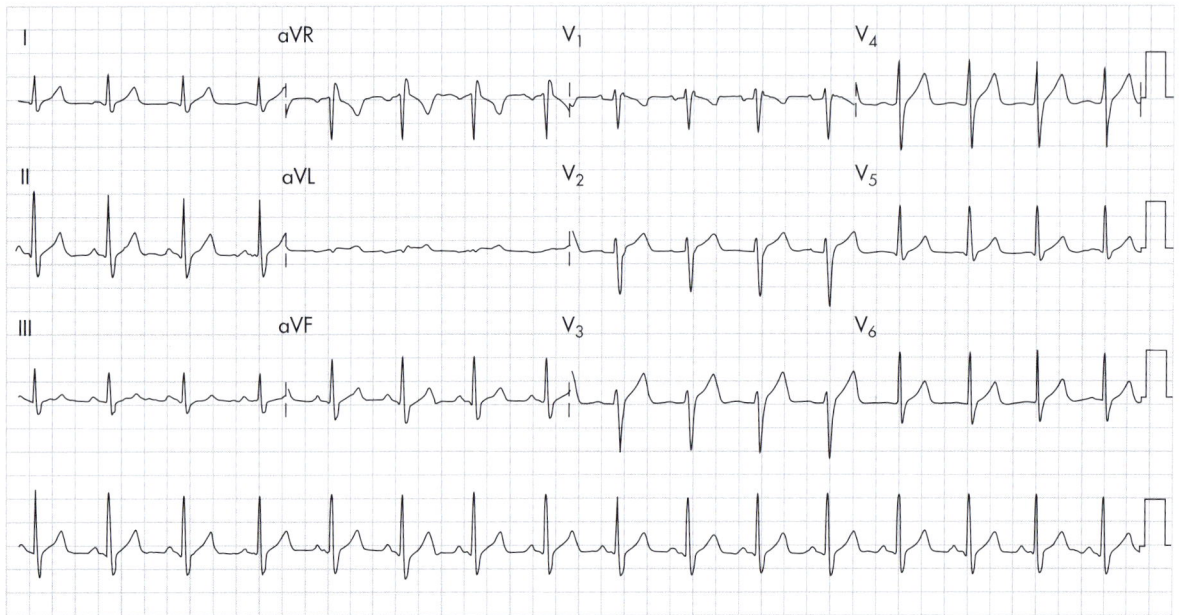

Figure 3.37a

CASE STUDY ON ECG 37

A 23-year-old East Asian man presented to emergency after an episode of syncope due to cardiac arrest. He was administered prompt cardiopulmonary resuscitation by a bystander. Paramedics found him to be in ventricular fibrillation. Prompt defibrillation had restored his pulse and the normal cardiac rhythm. He had been suffering from a febrile illness over the preceding two days. It was revealed that he has a family history of sudden death at a young age.

Please interpret the ECG in Figure 3.37a in a systematic manner.

Rhythm _____

Rate _____

Axis _____

P wave _____

PR interval _____

QRS complex _____

ST segment _____

T wave morphology _____

QT interval _____

Conclusion _____

Clinical notes _____

Diagnosis _____

_____

_____

_____

_____

Further investigations _____

_____

_____

_____

Management _____

_____

_____

_____

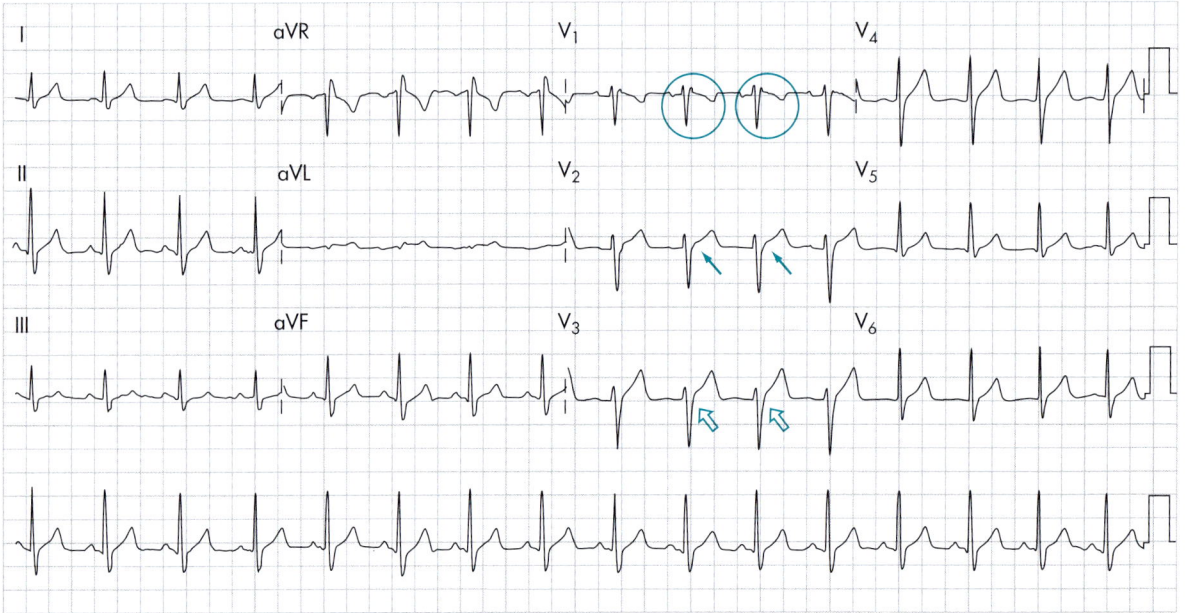

Figure 3.37b Brugada syndrome

ANSWER TO CASE STUDY ON ECG 37: BRUGADA SYNDROME

The ECG shows sinus rhythm at a rate of 100 bpm. The axis is normal (Fig 3.37b).

The most important changes are seen in leads V_1, V_2 and V_3. Lead V_1 shows an incomplete right bundle branch block (RBBB) pattern with a coved ST segment elevation of just over 1 mm and T wave inversion (circles). Lead V_2 shows ST segment elevation of about 2 mm (thin arrows). Lead V_3 shows ST segment elevation of 2 mm (thick arrows). All three leads show the J point elevation of approximately 2 mm.

These features are suggestive of Brugada syndrome (type 3).

The patient has a significant family history of sudden cardiac death, he is of East Asian origin and his ECG shows features suggestive of Brugada syndrome. These factors indicate the need for him to be managed with the implantation of a cardiac defibrillator.

Genetic inheritance of Brugada syndrome is complex. Several different genetic mutations have been described. The mutations affect the sodium channels in the heart; hence it is called a channelopathy. In addition to familial inheritance, Brugada syndrome can develop as a result of spontaneous new mutation too.

ECG characteristics can be seen at intermittent intervals. Challenging the patient with a sodium channel-blocking agent such as flecainide, procainamide or ajmaline can trigger these changes. Such challenge tests may help confirm the diagnosis.

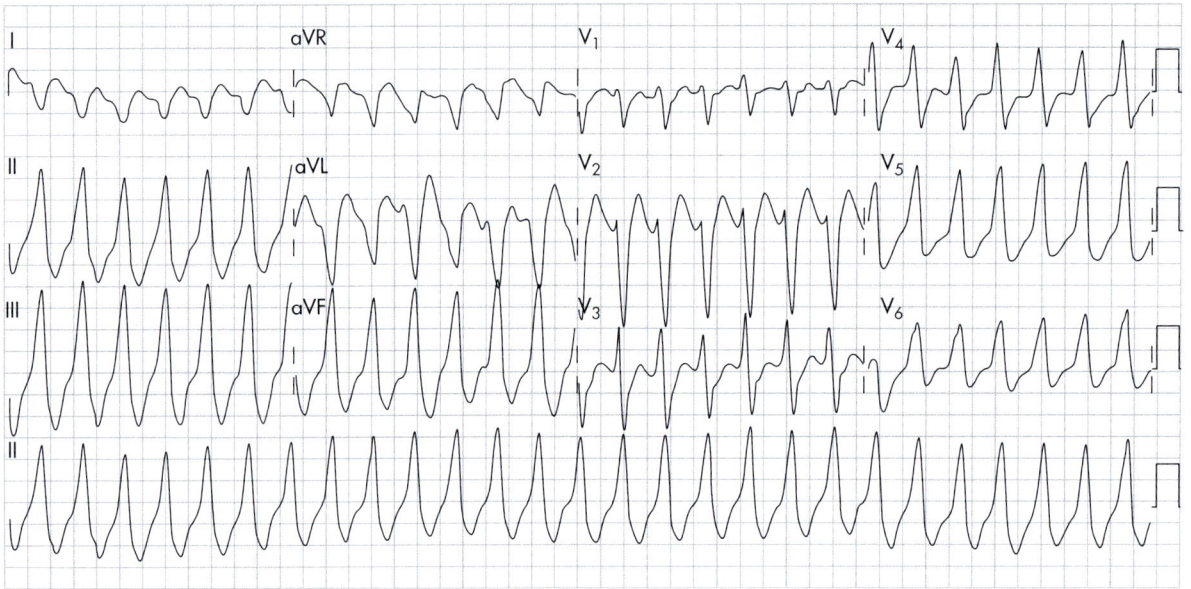

Figure 3.38a

CASE STUDY ON ECG 38

A 60-year-old female with a known history of coronary disease presents with chest pain. While being monitored in emergency this ECG was taken. The patient was complaining of feeling very light headed with a mean blood pressure of 44 mmHg.

Please interpret the ECG in Figure 3.38a in a systematic manner.

Rhythm _____

Rate _____

Axis _____

P wave _____

PR interval _____

QRS complex _____

ST segment _____

T wave morphology _____

QT interval _____

Conclusion _____

Clinical notes _____

Diagnosis _____

_____

_____

_____

_____

Further investigations _____

_____

_____

_____

_____

Management _____

_____

_____

_____

_____

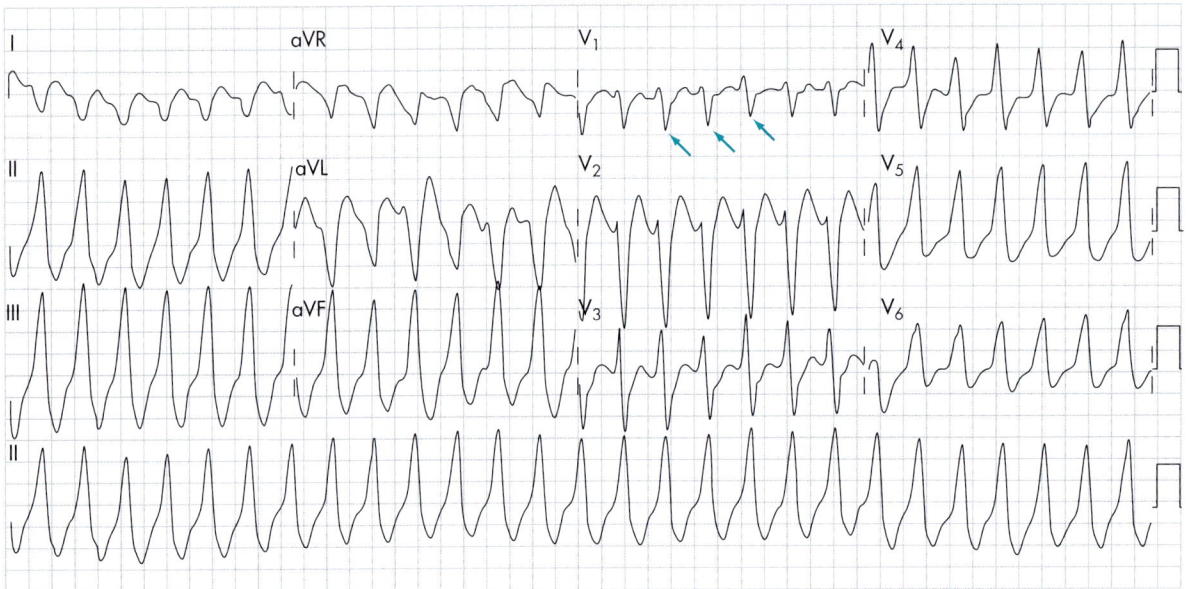

Figure 3.38b Ventricular tachycardia

ANSWER TO CASE STUDY ON ECG 38: VENTRICULAR TACHYCARDIA

Note that this is a regular tachycardia at a rate of 160 bpm (Fig 3.38b). Axis is deviated to the right (105°).

The QRS complex is very broad (>180 ms). There are left bundle branch block patterns in the QRS complexes in the precordial leads (V_1 to V_6). The QRS complex in V_1 is projected predominantly inferiorly (arrows).

This broad complex tachycardia is ventricular tachycardia (VT) due to the following reasons:

1 Patient has a known history of ischaemic heart disease

2 Patient is over the age of 35 years (VT is more common than supraventricular tachycardia (SVT)

3 A negative QRS complex in V_1 together with right axis deviation.

The diagnosis is sustained VT. The patient needs to be treated with DC electrical cardioversion upon rapid induction anaesthesia. Synchronised shock should be given if the patient has a pulse (pulseless VT is treated with defibrillation). She may require intravenous anti-arrhythmic therapy with amiodarone, procainamide or lignocaine. Intravenous magnesium is useful too.

Upon cardioversion she needs to be further investigated. Look for any QT interval prolongation in the ECG. Do an echocardiogram to look for heart failure. Non-invasive testing for coronary ischaemia should also be carried out. A long-term management plan will be based on the investigation findings. Long-term therapy will include amiodarone, beta-blockers and an implantable cardiac defibrillator.

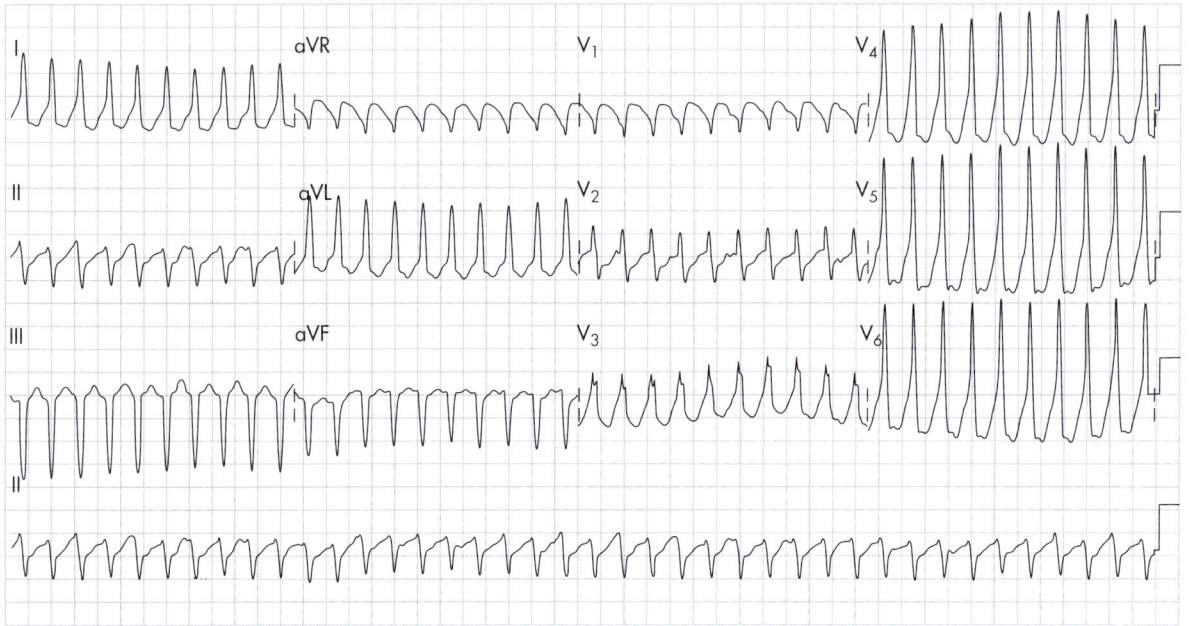

Figure 3.39a

CASE STUDY ON ECG 39

A 57-year-old woman presents with palpitations. She has a history of syncope. Upon further assessment an ECG was taken.

Please interpret the ECG in Figure 3.39a in a systematic manner.

Rhythm _____

Rate _____

Axis _____

P wave _____

PR interval _____

QRS complex _____

ST segment _____

T wave morphology _____

QT interval _____

Conclusion _____

Clinical notes _____

Diagnosis _____

_____

_____

_____

_____

Further investigations _____

_____

_____

_____

Management _____

_____

_____

_____

_____

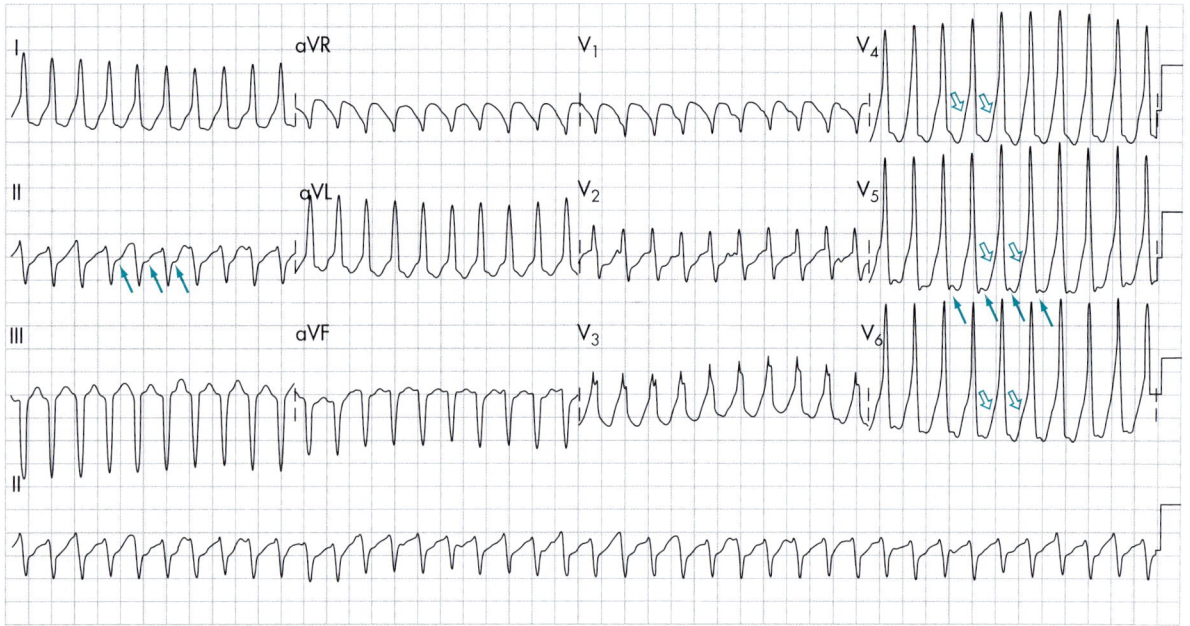

Figure 3.39b Supraventricular tachycardia

ANSWER TO CASE STUDY ON ECG 39: SUPRAVENTRICULAR TACHYCARDIA

A

Note that this is a regular tachycardia at a rate of 240 bpm (Fig 3.39b). The axis is to the right (right axis deviation (RAD)).

The QRS complex duration is 110 ms. Note the retrograde P waves appearing just after the QRS complex (thin arrows).

The RP interval is shorter than the RR interval.

The QRS complex is narrower than 120 ms indicating that this is a supraventricular tachycardia.

Note the slurred first part of the QRS complex indicating the presence of a delta wave (thick arrows). This represents conduction via the accessory atrioventricular pathway.

This is likely to be atrioventricular reentrant tachycardia (AVRT) due to Wolff-Parkinson-White syndrome.

Management should include initial vagal manoeuvres to slow the heart rate and possibly terminate the arrhythmia. If these measures fail, adenosine injection should be tried. Vagal manoeuvres or an adenosine injection should only be done with the defibrillator on stand by. If medical therapy fails, the patient may require DC electrical cardioversion. She may need referral to an electrophysiologist to map the accessory pathway by performing an electrophysiological study. This accessory pathway can then be ablated with radiofrequency energy thus effectively curing her of the condition.

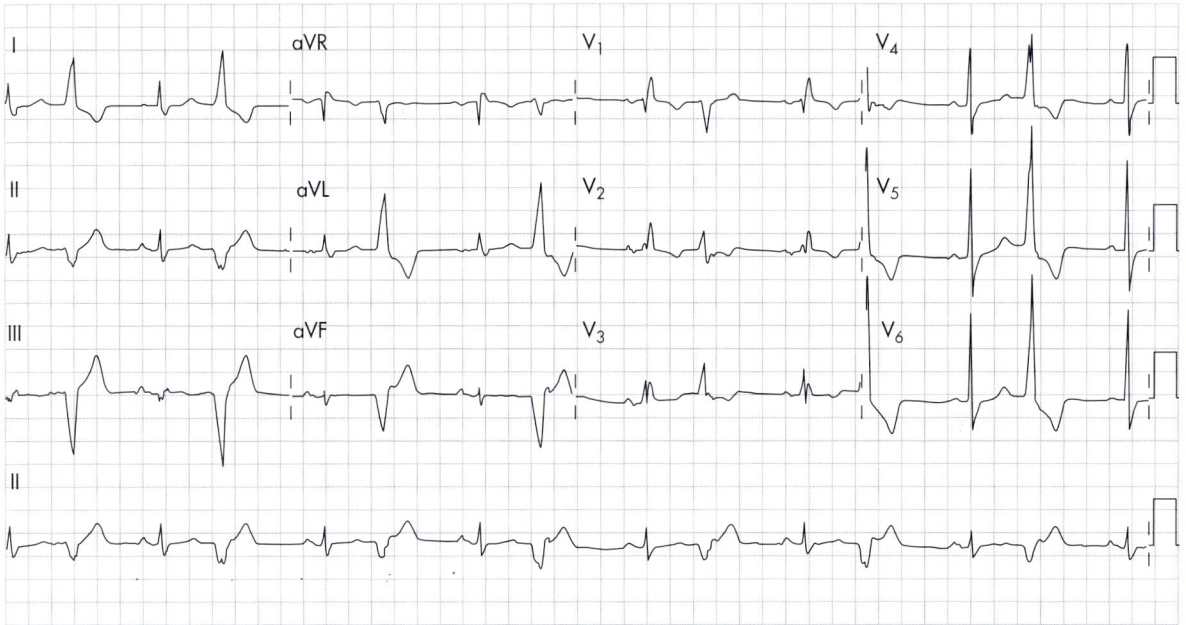

Figure 3.40a

CASE STUDY ON ECG 40

Q

This 49-year-old man presents with palpitations. He was anxious. An ECG recording was obtained in the assessment.

Please interpret the ECG in Figure 3.40a in a systematic manner.

Rhythm _____

Rate _____

Axis _____

P wave _____

PR interval _____

QRS complex _____

ST segment _____

T wave morphology _____

QT interval _____

Conclusion _____

Clinical notes _____

Diagnosis _____

_____

_____

_____

_____

Further investigations _____

_____

_____

_____

_____

Management _____

_____

_____

_____

_____

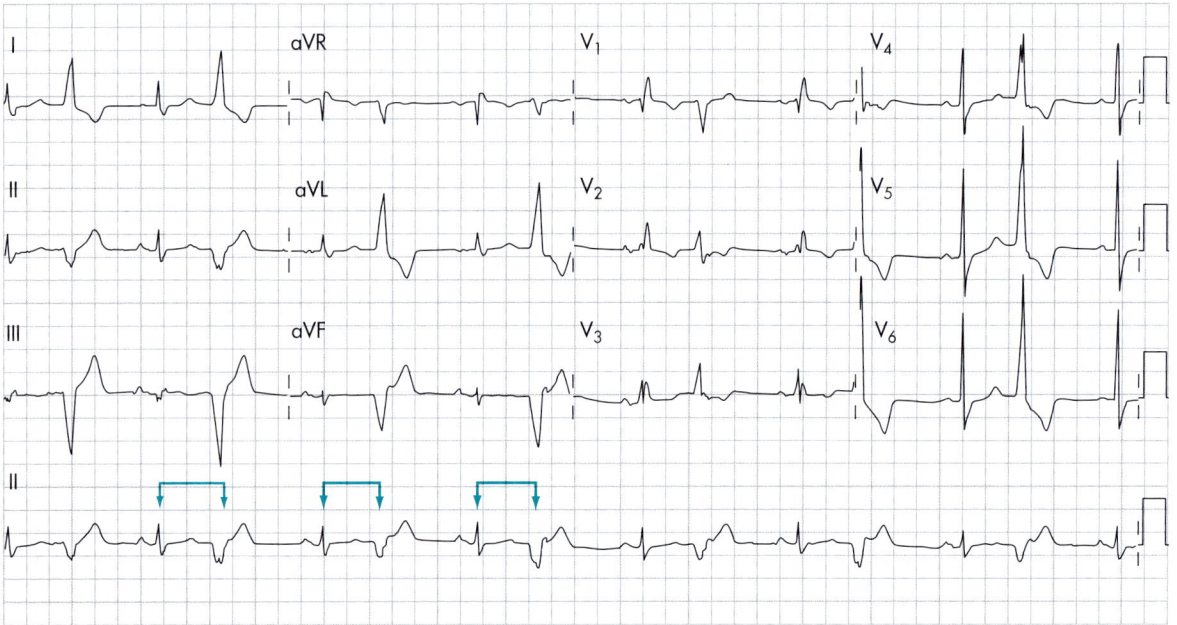

Figure 3.40b Ventricular bigeminy

ANSWER TO CASE STUDY ON ECG 40: VENTRICULAR BIGEMINY

The rate is approximately 100 bpm. The rhythm is regularly irregular (Fig 3.40b).

Note the native sinus QRS complexes of narrower morphology. The axis of these complexes remains within normal limits.

The native complexes show a right bundle branch block pattern.

A wide QRS complex of ventricular origin accompanies each native complex (paired arrows). Given the regular nature of it and its constant relationship to the sinus beat, this is called ventricular bigeminy.

The patient needs to be investigated for metabolic abnormalities by performing serum biochemistry tests. An echocardiogram is indicated to look for any structural heart disorder. Non-invasive testing for coronary ischaemia is indicated. If no underlying pathology is identified the patient can be reassured and managed conservatively.

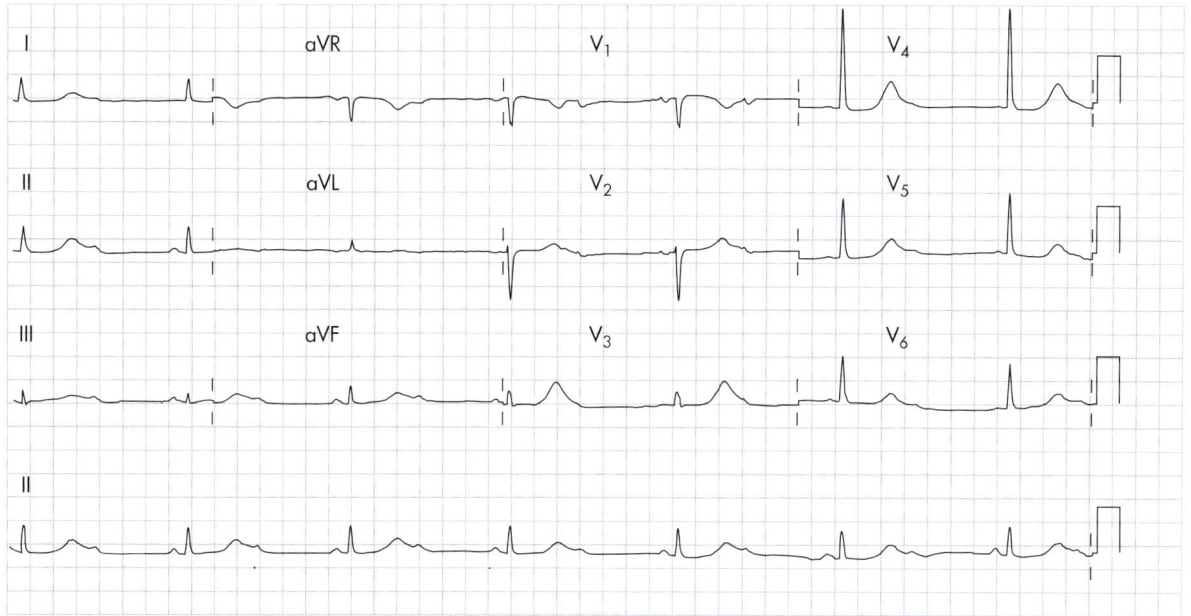

Figure 3.41a

CASE STUDY ON ECG 41

This 75-year-old man presents with fatigue and light headedness. During the assessment an ECG was obtained.

Please interpret the ECG in Figure 3.41a in a systematic manner.

Rhythm _____

Rate _____

Axis _____

P wave _____

PR interval _____

QRS complex _____

ST segment _____

T wave morphology _____

QT interval _____

Conclusion _____

Clinical notes _____

Diagnosis _____

_____

_____

_____

_____

Further investigations _____

_____

_____

_____

Management _____

_____

_____

_____

_____

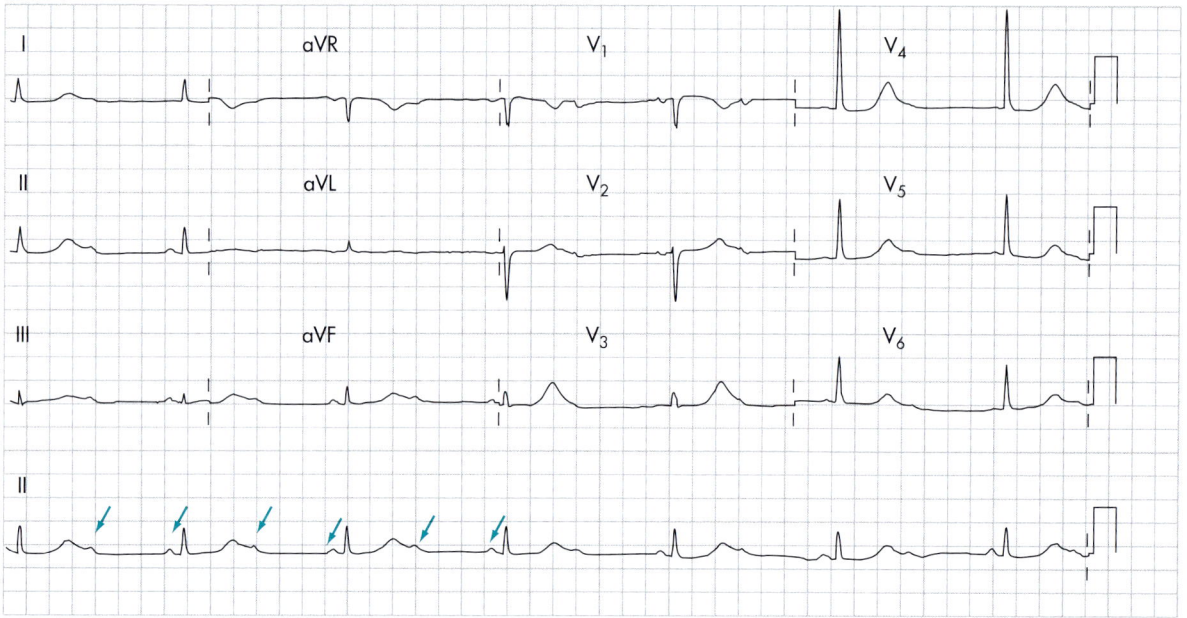

Figure 3.41b Second degree heart block

ANSWER TO CASE STUDY ON ECG 41: SECOND DEGREE HEART BLOCK

A

The rhythm is regular. Note that the rate is 40 bpm indicating bradycardia (Fig 3.41b). Axis is normal.

The most striking abnormality is that for every two P waves (arrows) only one is followed by a QRS complex. The PR interval in the conducted beats remains within normal limits. This is Mobitz type II second degree heart block.

Second degree heart block has two types:

1 Mobitz type I second degree heart block (Wenckebach phenomenon) is where the PR interval gradually gets longer till one P wave fails to conduct to the ventricle. This is due to a conduction defect in the AV node and is a benign phenomenon.

2 Mobitz type II second degree heart block is due to a conduction defect that is located inferior to the AV node in the vicinity of the bundle of His. This conduction defect can progress to complete heart block. If no causative factor is identified, such as reversible coronary ischaemia or a medication that blocks cardiac conduction, the patient needs to be treated with the implantation of a permanent pacemaker.

This patient should be assessed for any reversible cause for the heart block. If none is found he needs to be treated with the implantation of a permanent pacemaker.

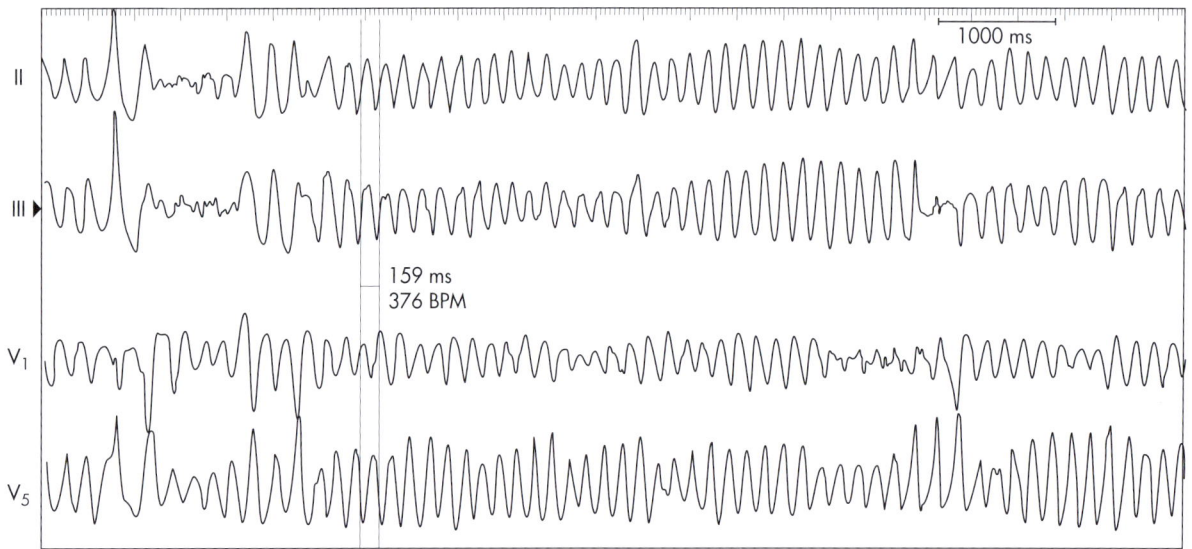

Figure 3.42a

CASE STUDY ON ECG 42

This 37-year-old man presented with an episode of syncope. His medication history included clarithromycin for a recent respiratory tract infection. While in emergency he had another episode where he felt very dizzy and then rapidly passed out. The ECG monitor captured the rhythm during the episode.

Please interpret the ECG in Figure 3.42a in a systematic manner.

Rhythm _____

Rate _____

Axis _____

P wave _____

PR interval _____

QRS complex _____

ST segment _____

T wave morphology _____

QT interval _____

Conclusion _____

Clinical notes _____

Diagnosis _____

_____

_____

_____

_____

Further investigations _____

_____

_____

_____

Management _____

_____

_____

_____

_____

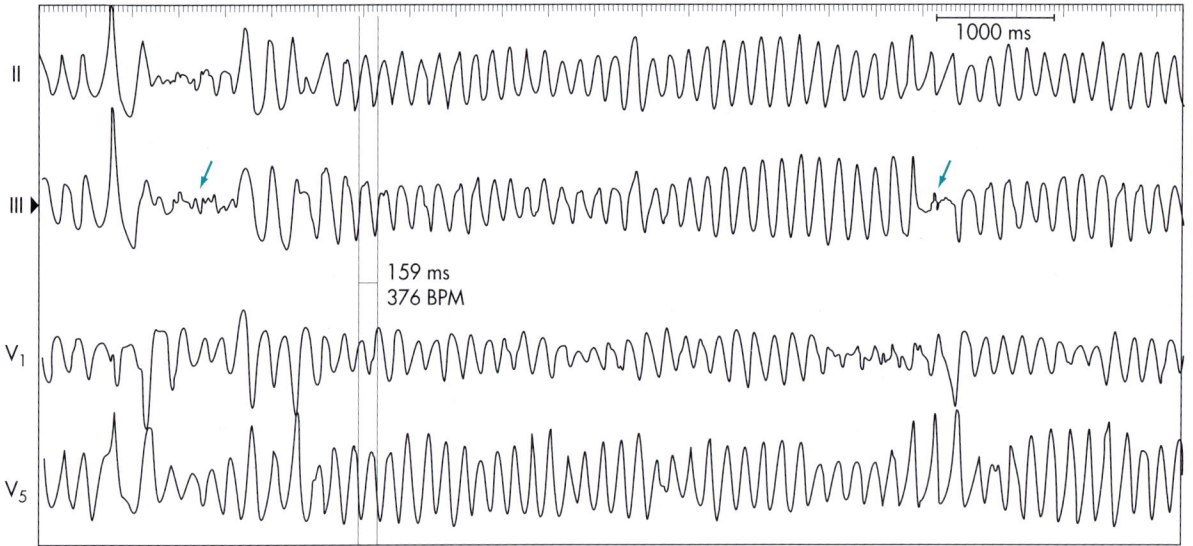

Figure 3.42b Torsades de pointes VT

ANSWER TO CASE STUDY ON ECG 42: TORSADES DE POINTES VT

A

This is a broad complex tachycardia at a rate close to 300 bpm (Fig 3.42b). The axis shifts between the right side and the left side. You can appreciate that the axis shifts its direction repeatedly by at least 180°.

Note the classic spindle shape of the ECG tracings. The QRS complex morphology changes between beats, hence it is called polymorphic VT.

This is torsades de pointes (twisting of the points) ventricular tachycardia.

Also note occasional capture beats (arrows) representing conducted sinus beats.

This man needs to be treated with prompt defibrillation. His subsequent resting ECG may show a very prolonged QT interval due to clarithromycin. Upon cessation of this agent the QT interval may normalise.

If the patient is in haemodynamic compromise immediate DC electrical cardioversion or defibrillation is indicated. Torsades can degenerate to VF.

Other therapies in the setting of torsades include:

- Parenteral magnesium
- Isoprenaline infusion
- Overdrive pacing with a temporary pacing wire insertion
- Anti-arrhythmic agents such as mexiletine.

These measures are indicated if the patient is haemodynamically stable.

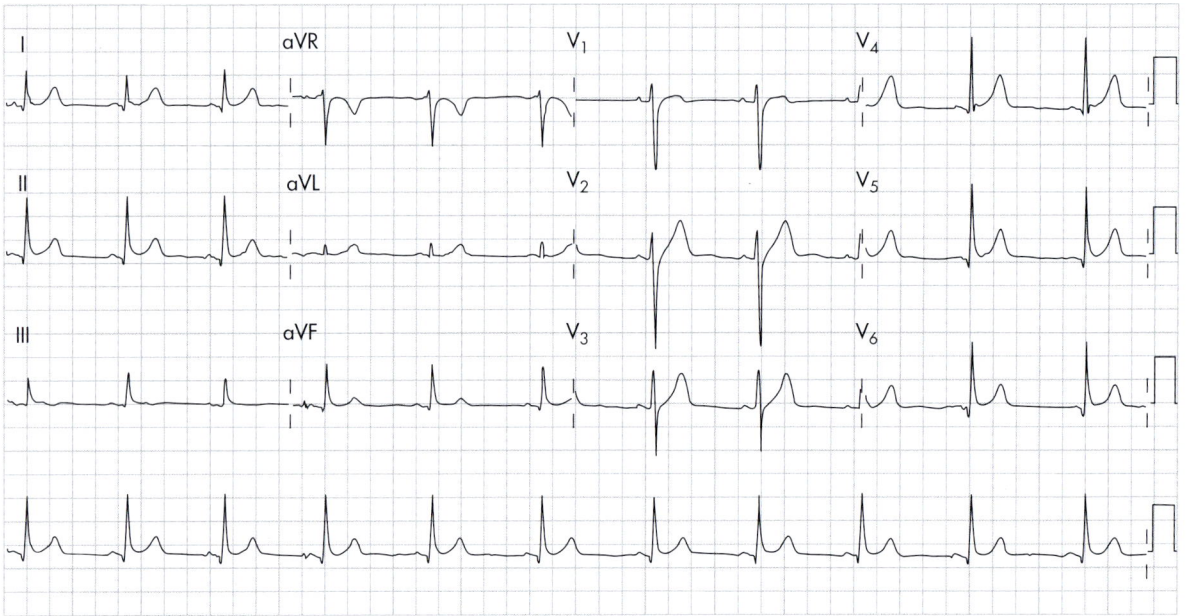

Figure 3.43a

CASE STUDY ON ECG 43

A 25-year-old man presents with sharp left-sided chest pain that worsens on inspiration and leaning forward. On examination a friction rub was audible over the precordium. An ECG was taken subsequently.

Please interpret the ECG in Figure 3.43a in a systematic manner.

Rhythm _____

Rate _____

Axis _____

P wave _____

PR interval _____

QRS complex _____

ST segment _____

T wave morphology _____

QT interval _____

Conclusion _____

Clinical notes _____

Diagnosis _____

_____

_____

_____

_____

Further investigations _____

_____

_____

_____

_____

Management _____

_____

_____

_____

_____

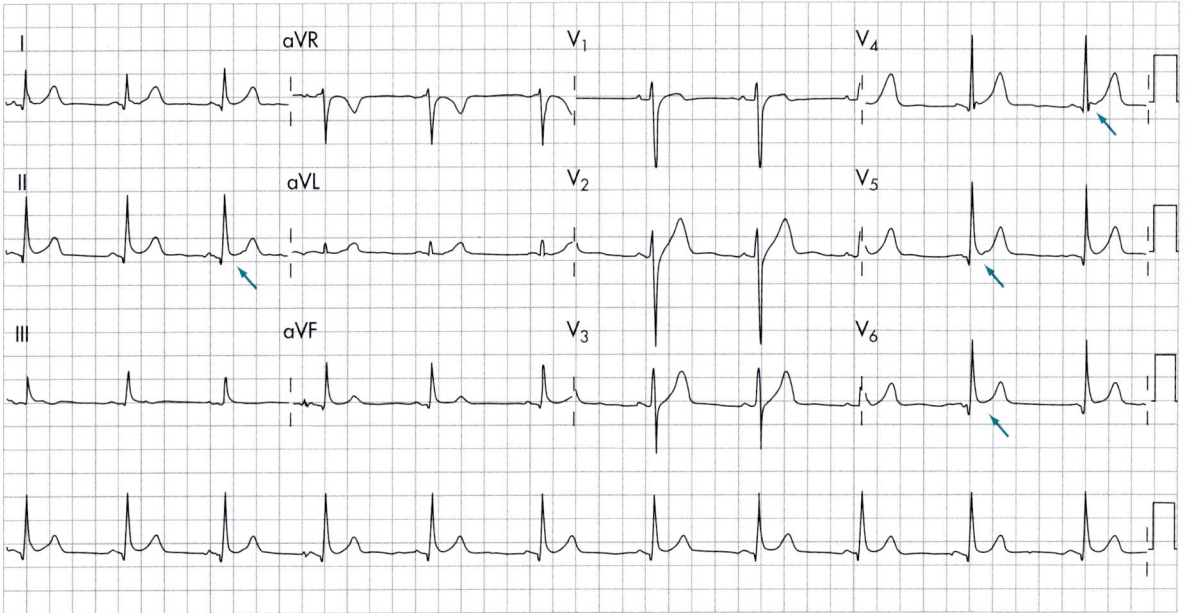

Figure 3.43b Acute pericarditis

ANSWER TO CASE STUDY ON ECG 43: ACUTE PERICARDITIS

The rate is 65 bpm and the rhythm is regular (Fig 3.43b). The axis is within normal limits at 56°.

The significant abnormality is the concave-up ST segment elevation seen in multiple leads (arrows). There is very subtle PR depression seen in leads II and aVF.

The clinical picture and the ECG changes are very suggestive of acute pericarditis.

The patient may benefit from echocardiography to exclude pericardial effusion that sometimes accompanies pericarditis. His full blood count, electrolyte profile and renal function should be checked.

The most common cause of acute pericarditis is a viral infection. The patient needs to be treated with a non-steroidal antiinflammatory agent for a short period until the symptoms fully settle.

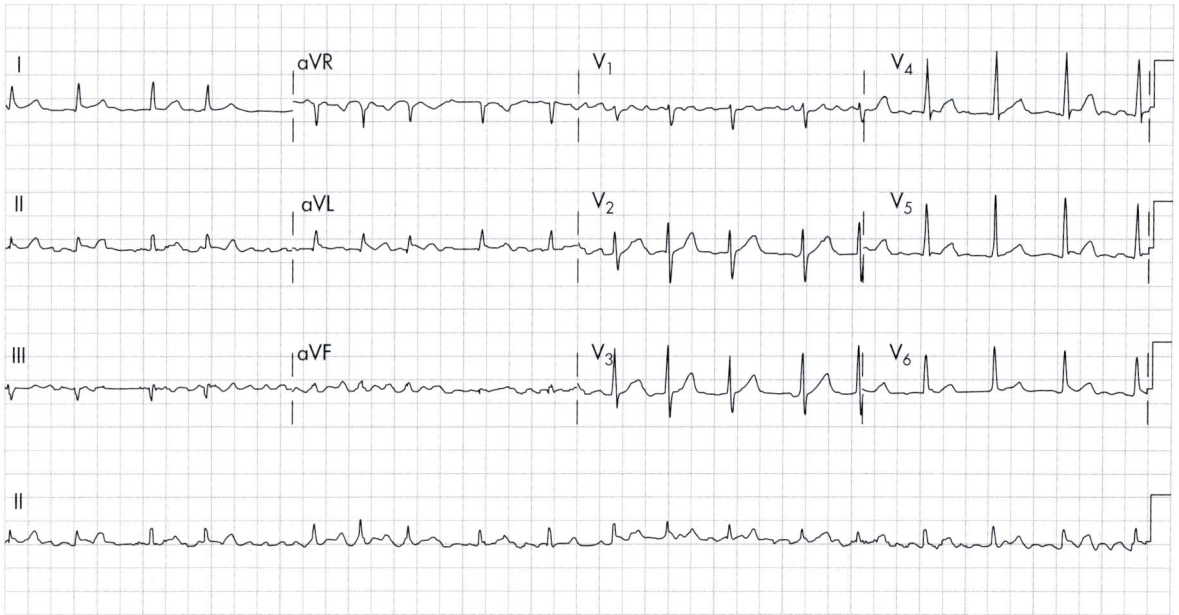

Figure 3.44a

CASE STUDY ON ECG 44

This 40-year-old man presents with light headedness. He has been unwell for almost a week. He could remember experiencing severe sharp chest pain about a week ago that was relieved by antiinflammatory drugs given by his general practitioner. He is otherwise well. On examination he had distended neck veins, a positive Kussmaul's sign and hypotension with pulsus paradoxes. His ECG is as shown.

Please interpret the ECG in Figure 3.44a in a systematic manner.

Rhythm _____

Rate _____

Axis _____

P wave _____

PR interval _____

QRS complex _____

ST segment _____

T wave morphology _____

QT interval _____

Conclusion _____

Clinical notes _____

Diagnosis _____

_____

_____

_____

Further investigations _____

_____

_____

_____

Management _____

_____

_____

_____

_____

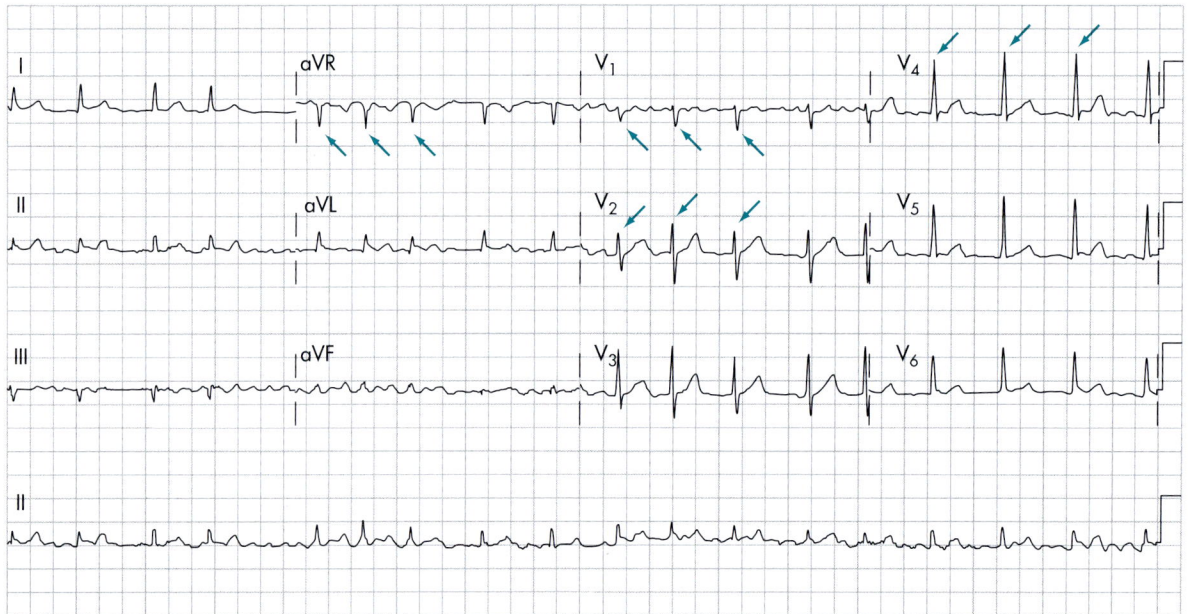

Figure 3.44b Pericardial effusion and voltage alternans

ANSWER TO CASE STUDY ON ECG 44: PERICARDIAL EFFUSION AND ELECTRICAL ALTERNANS

A

The rhythm is irregularly irregular. The rate varies between 110 and 140 bpm. The axis is 17° and normal (Fig 3.44b).

The QRS complex is narrow at 76 ms and the QT interval is normal for the rate.

The significant findings are:

1 The small size of the QRS complexes — these are also called low voltage complexes.

2 The changing amplitude of the QRS complexes, particularly in the precordial and lateral leads (arrows). This is called electrical alternans or voltage alternans.

These features are highly suggestive of a large pericardial effusion. Electrical alternans is due to the heart 'floating' and 'wobbling' within the over-filled pericardial reservoir. Due to this wobbling the cardiac axis shifts repeatedly.

The ECG diagnosis is consistent with the physical findings of cardiac tamponade, such as Kussmaul's sign in the jugular venous pulse (rise in jugular venous pulse (JVP) on inspiration)

and pulsus paradoxes (systolic pressure drop of over 10 mmHg on inspiration).

This patient needs urgent echocardiogram to confirm the diagnosis. Pericardial fluid should be drained by emergency pericardiocentesis. Once drained the fluid collection should be sent for pathological analysis.

The most likely scenario is that the patient may have suffered from acute viral pericarditis in the preceding week. As the inflammation settled, a pericardial effusion has rapidly accumulated. This is not an uncommon sequel to acute pericarditis. Blood tests may show elevated inflammatory markers such as ESR and CRP.

The AF with rapid ventricular response may be a reaction to the acute illness. AF may revert to sinus rhythm once the acute illness settles. However if AF persists consider rate control or rhythm control therapy.

The patient's thyroid function indices should be checked as thyroid disease too can cause AF as well as pericardial effusion.

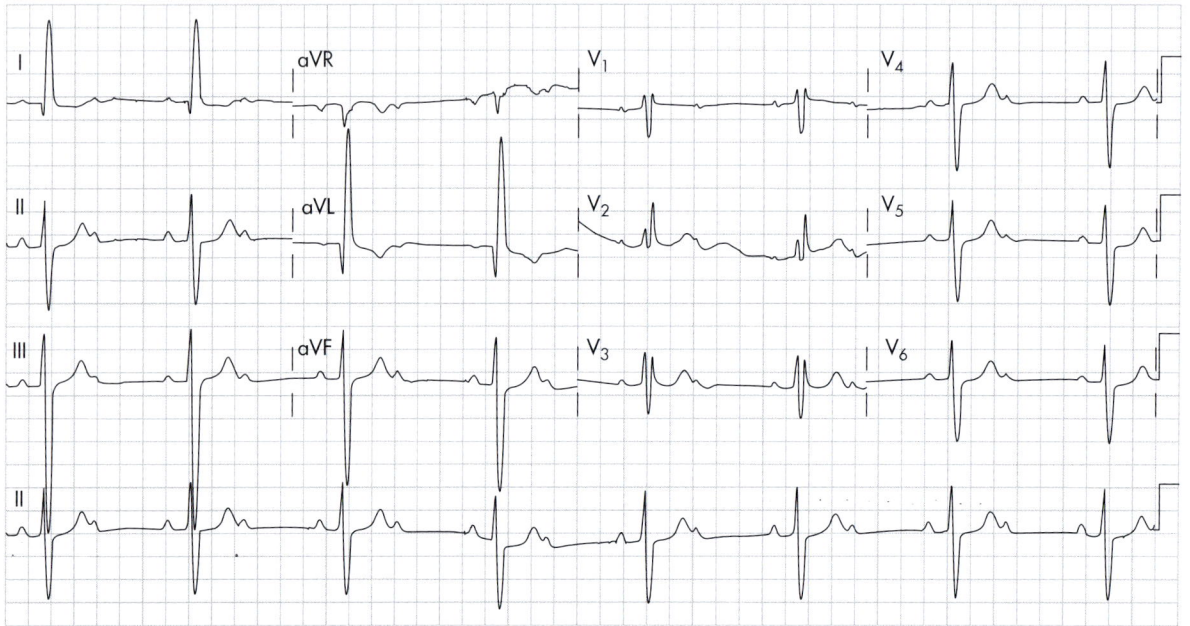

Figure 3.45a

CASE STUDY ON ECG 45

This 75-year-old man presents with light headedness. He has a history of chronic lung disease and hypertension. Upon further assessment this ECG was obtained.

Please interpret the ECG in Figure 3.45a in a systematic manner.

Rhythm _____

Rate _____

Axis _____

P wave _____

PR interval _____

QRS complex _____

ST segment _____

T wave morphology _____

QT interval _____

Conclusion _____

Clinical notes _____

Diagnosis _____

_____

_____

_____

_____

Further investigations _____

_____

_____

_____

_____

Management _____

_____

_____

_____

_____

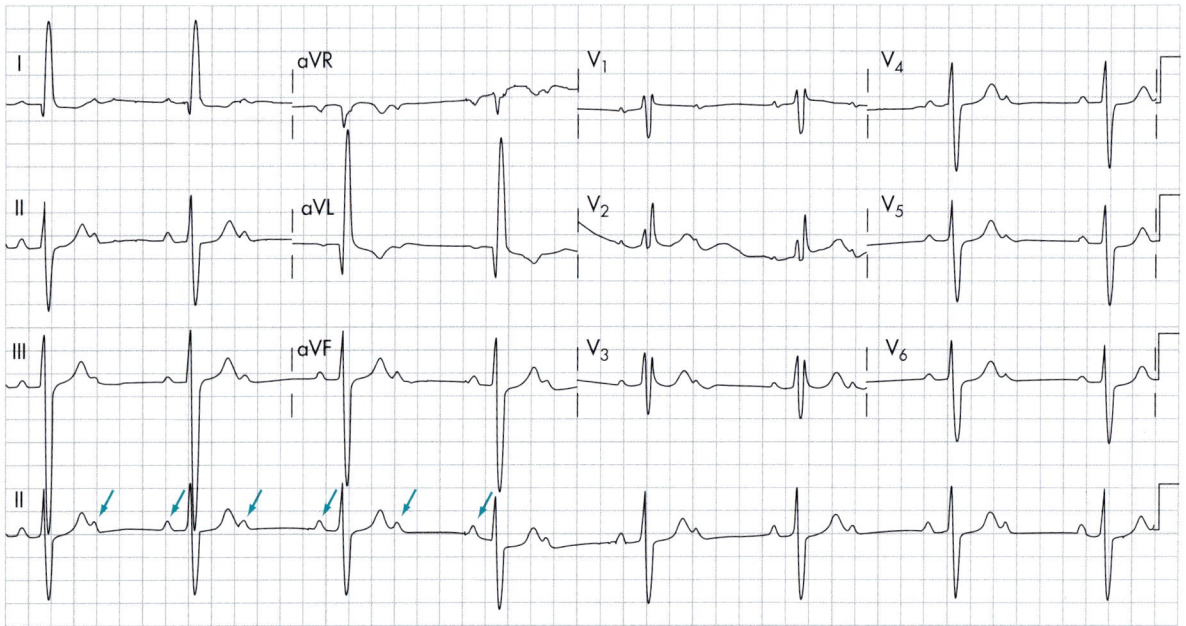

Figure 3.45b Extensive conduction defects

ANSWER TO CASE STUDY ON ECG 45: EXTENSIVE CONDUCTION DEFECTS

A

This ECG shows sinus rhythm and bradycardia at 45 bpm (Fig 3.45b). The axis is −45° and deviated to the left.

Only one out of two P waves is followed by a QRS complex (arrows). This means that only one out of every two P waves is conducted to the ventricle. This is type II second degree heart block.

The QRS complex is prolonged (133 ms).

QRS morphology is suggestive of right bundle branch block with rSr pattern in lead V_1 and deep S wave seen in lead V_6. This is not the typical RBBB pattern where the R wave should be more prominent in lead V_1.

Tall R waves are seen in the lateral leads (leads I and aVL) indicating left ventricular hypertrophy.

This man's extensive cardiac conduction defects should be treated with the implantation of a permanent pacemaker.

He needs to be further investigated with echocardiography to confirm the diagnosis of left ventricular hypertrophy. His hypertension needs to be controlled aggressively to prevent further progression of hypertensive heart disease.

Appendix
NYHA Functional Class

The New York Heart Association (NYHA) functional class is used to describe the level of effort that is tolerated by a patient with heart failure. NYHA classification is useful in deciding on the optimal management of the heart failure. In addition, the NYHA class can predict the patient's overall prognosis.

The NYHA classification is as follows:

Class 1 — Patient does not feel breathless with ordinary activity (i.e. walking to the shops)

Class 2 — Mildly breathless on ordinary activity

Class 3 — Symptomatic/breathless with minimal activity (i.e. walking to the toilet)

Class 4 — Symptomatic/breathless at rest.

Index

Page numbers followed by "f" indicate figures, "t" indicate tables, and "b" indicate boxes.

➡